Back to Life

Back
to
Life

Introducing the Simple Cure for Back Pain and Sitting Ills

S.E.E.D.

(Seven Essential Exercises Daily)

Condict Moore, M.D.

B
Butler
Books

For my children and grandchildren,
hoping they may find a path to
longer and more rewarding life than
previous generations.

Published in the USA by
BUTLER BOOKS
P.O. Box 7311
Louisville, KY 40207

Printed in Canada

ISBN 1-884532-52-7

Many persons have taken time to respond to me about their experiences with these exercises. Their support gave me confidence to write the book; to them I am grateful.

Outstanding skill and commitment fortunately came my way from the following individuals: my daughter, Carrie Moore, original drawing artist; Vera Strohbeck, my office right hand for over 30 years; David Hartman, gifted designer; Denise Eberhart, accomplished printer; Martha Neal Cooke, book marketer supreme; Robert Schulman, noted journalist and friend; Keith Runyon, *Courier-Journal* editor; Tommy Smith, top golf club professional; Donald M. Miller, M.D., leading medical innovator; Helyn Jenkins, skillful proofreader; and my wife, Caroline, superb critic and my life sustainer.

CONTENTS

Chapter 1 – How Back Recovery Began, 9

Chapter 2 – Health Progress Seems Stalled, 15

Chapter 3 – Our Sitting Existence, 29

Chapter 4 – How Sitting Hurts Us, 35

Chapter 5 – Solving the Sitting Problem, 45

Chapter 6 – The Seven Essential Exercises Daily (SEED), 49

Chapter 7 – Dailyness, 71

Chapter 8 – One Person's Experience With SEED, 73

Chapter 9 – Who Needs SEED, 77

Chapter 10 – Measuring SEED Progress, 87

Chapter 11 – Questions and Answers, 91

Chapter 12 – Breathing As Exercise, 97

Chapter 13 – On Back Pain, 101

Chapter 14 – Attention Computer Users, 105

Chapter 15 – Improved Golf With SEED, 107

Chapter 16 – The Exercises and Sex, 111

Chapter 17 – The Exercises and Travel, 115

Chapter 18 – The Family Habit, 119

Chapter 19 – The Early Disability Syndrome, 123

Chapter 20 – The Seven Exercises and Aging, 129

Chapter 21 – The Case for Sitting, 133

Chapter 22 – My Predictions, 137

Chapter 23 – In Conclusion, 141

Readings, 144

Chapter 1 ⎯⎯⎯⎯⎯⎯⎯⎯⎯⎯⎯⎯
HOW BACK RECOVERY BEGAN

When I reached the age of 70 I knew I had to retire from cancer surgery. I was getting too tired standing for hours each day at the operating table. I just couldn't function at top level anymore.

I had no idea what I'd do in retirement. I decided to keep open a small part-time office to see old patients in consultation, mostly those who had survived cancer. Also, I expected to have some time to recover my golf game, which had lapsed into dufferdom during working years.

I was glad to feel less tired. However, as time went on, one thing stopped my recreation—my back hurt a lot. The more I swung the golf club, the more pain I got. I had back pain every morning. I thought, what kind of retirement was this? I had been fairly active all my life and had had some back pain attacks like everybody else, but now, when I quit the heavy stress of daily surgery, my back got worse.

Like everybody else with back pain, I went to chiropractors, took anti-inflammatory drugs, used magnetic belts, sacroiliac belts, and back braces. I consulted with my orthopedic friends, got x-rays, received the diagnosis of "facetitis" but no definitive treatment except rest. I took injections at spine clinics, saw physiotherapists, went to gym workouts and back specialty stores. My back still hurt. I studied exercise books, watched tapes, reviewed an elaborate array of popular fitness programs and machines (a multi-billion dollar business). Of course, I tried the pain-killers of the day—they either didn't agree with me or wore thin.

I talked with many friends about low back pain. It seems everybody had it. Everybody had a pet remedy, but nothing permanently abolished pain for me. What was going on? I became fixated with the great irony of it all—everybody had back pain, but all of modern medicine and sports authorities couldn't find a lasting remedy.

Finally, after many months of unsatisfactory results, I began experimenting on my own with some home calisthenics related to low back structural anatomy. I concentrated on the lower back because that's where it hurt. I was careful to rest for two weeks until my pain subsided enough so that any small tears could heal and joint inflammation could subside.

After daily floor stretching, turning and deep breathing, each day I began to feel better. I observed that loosening my lower back with gradual daily exercises made it feel healthy.

That was curious: people I had talked to previously felt (as I myself did) that keeping a stiff lower back was beneficial—this explained the braces, pads, avoidance of bending, etc., to which we all resorted. Now I saw clearly that it was the reverse—gradual mobilization of stiff lower back joints restored normal function without pain. Immobility would not cure my back; mobility would.

With this conclusion, I was off to the races finally. I tested and refined and selected and practiced various lower back looseners until I had a simple set of seven basic exercises that kept my back pain-free despite a full golf swing. Now the question was, would this hold up?

I am glad to report that it has held up for 17 years now. I have no back pain. I am as active as I can be at my age. But I do wonder why I am not degenerating faster, like my contemporaries are doing.

After several years of doing my floor calisthenics and marveling at their efficacy, and prompted by many friends who were interested in my regime, I coined a name for it—the Seven Essential Exercises Daily, or SEED for short. I took it upon myself to print a little booklet illustrating the exercises and began giving it out to friends and anyone who inquired, and pretty soon I was going through them at a good clip. Then, a year or so ago, the local newspaper got wind of my back routine and printed an article about it, which I reprint below:

LIFETIME FITNESS FOR EVERYONE
By Condict Moore, M.D.

After spending a lifetime in modern medicine, I have tumbled to an astonishing fact; humans are only living a few years longer today than they did in biblical times. The Bible records a life expectancy of "three score years and ten" (70 years).

We can do better than an additional five years in two millennia. Science estimates we could live at least 100 years; 60,000 Americans already have done it.

In a broad historical view of our civilization's progress, two changes stand out:

People now sit inactive most of their waking hours, and, with plenty of food, eat more than they need; people used to exert themselves continually, as humans are constructed to do, mainly to get enough food.

The diseases that carry people off before their time today are the degenerative, "decay" type of diseases like diabetes, heart disease, obesity, arthritis, osteoporosis, cancer and the dementias (Alzheimer's). They are not new ailments, but their early onset and frequency are new in the last 50 years.

To my medical mind, a lifetime of sitting that crunches our vital organs and systems, cramps and slows our repair mechanisms by hurting circulation, respiration, immune responses and endocrine effects and feed-backs in body and brain, where easy eating is the popular pleasure--all of this can easily cause a hastening of the natural bodily decay schedule by 20 or 25 years.

What we are doing to reverse this inactivity-chronic disease trend is not working. Sports are for the young; aerobics is for heart-disease prevention and rehab; walking is too mild and unfocused.

As I grow older, I am looking into this inaction -overeating-decay connection in order to try to live past 75. By experimenting with my own body in a minimal exercise program I have discovered several things of interest:

1) It requires action every day to counteract prolonged sitting--a few days a week, or exercise, be it intense or mild, when convenient, doesn't get the job done. 2) The major damage inflicted by prolonged daily sitting occurs to our backs, our spines, spinal-attached muscles and joints and damage to mid-section functions. 3) Daily back conditioning with measured deep breathing does wonders for back pains, posture, mobility, appetite regulation and mood. 4)A set of seven floor calisthenics can effect a vital recovery from sitting in only a few minutes each day.

Now, at 86 years of age, I am unhampered by "decay" diseases; I work and play as when younger, only slower. I do the seven essential exercises daily (SEED) and have for 15 years. They take only 13 minutes to perform with no gadgets or outside help. Thay make me feel good, keep my weight steady, my posture and mobility normal and my desire to live at a high.

As a real proof of their validity, I cite that my spouse does them eagerly every day. People will say I'm just lucky; no one will ever know the reason for my good health for sure. But I like to remember what Jack Nicklaus said when congratulated as lucky for making a fabulous golf shot: 'Thank you. And the more I practice the more luckier I get.'

Hundreds of my acquaintances enjoy SEED. I will send a descriptive booklet to anyone who wishes to begin. Write: Condict Moore, M.D., University of Louisville Brown Cancer Center, 529 S. Jackson St., Louisville, KY 40202. (One per person or family).

The above article was published in the Louisville *Courier-Journal*, July 7, 2002.

I didn't really expect many readers to ask for a booklet. To my surprise, I received over 1,100 requests. In the next few months they climbed to nearly 2,000. Over one hundred individuals so far have reported their experiences with the routine SEED to me in some detail. Virtually all expressed delight and were continuing with SEED daily.

This somewhat overwhelming response to one small item in the paper revealed to me a pent-up appetite for a refresher and restorer of physical function and feeling of well-being. I have been, therefore, encouraged to write this book to expand on SEED as part of 21st century living, mainly because many people seem to want it and to enjoy it.

Chapter 2 _____
HEALTH PROGRESS SEEMS STALLED

We modern humans don't live as long as we could or should. We have made great progress in this direction over the last century but the pace of progress now seems stalled.

Average longevity stood near 50 years of age in the 19th century; it now stands at around 75 years, which is a good 50% increase. At this rate we should average 100 years of life by the end of 2100 A.D. But I don't believe it will happen for two reasons:

1) Past progress was relatively easy. Bad sanitation, acute germ diseases that kill, food scarcity, infant mortality and serious injuries all responded to and were ameliorated by medical science, which identified specific causes and devised clear-cut cures;

2) The chronic death-dealers that prevail today, like heart disease, stroke, cancer, dementia, obesity and several less common ailments, do not have specific, single causes; they are only partially helped by modern treatments. These chronic ailments that impede

15

the public's longevity are coming on us at earlier ages and advancing more rapidly than in the past. Our gains, therefore, are getting cancelled out. At this rate we'll be lucky to average 85 years of age by 2100 A.D.

No doubt exists that we *can* live for 100 years. Sixty thousand Americans have already done it. Nature always provides an excess capacity for essential functions. In evolutionary terms, an extra 50 years of life potential for safety would not surprise a biologist. The reason average people don't live that long are multiple and still unclear, but one fact seems established—our longevity after the age of 50, after reproductive years are over, is not hard-wired into our genes. Evolution, which selects for survival, doesn't care much what happens after breeding and child-rearing have occurred. After we have offspring and raise them, nature leaves us alone. Whatever we do after that age is not determined by genetic inheritance, it is mostly from habits that we formed earlier. So the chronic diseases that cut short our natural decay are controllable.

Evolution may seem controversial; for some it threatens religious faith. But it has one great positive benefit—it can lead us to winnow out the parts of our behavior pattern that are hard-wired into our genes from the parts that are only "soft-wired" into our lives, the habits that we can change.

Habit and Genes

Confusion and ignorance about habit and genetic behavior abounds in our society. Today most people lump habitual behavior into the genetically-determined, hard-wired category. Specifically, if they don't like what's happening to them in older age, or can't understand it, they blame it on their genes—their inevitable inherited makeup which is not subject to change. In this way people ease themselves out of making much effort to change. "It won't make much difference in the long run how we live anyway," is the thinking.

This difference between genes and habit seems to me crucial. It represents the difference between the inevitable and the changeable, the problems we can't affect and the ones we can, the life dilemmans where there is no hope and the ones where there is real hope.

After 50 we are in the habit-determined, changable realm. In fact, our idea of seeing life as genetically engineered is a habit itself which continues to dominate our thinking when we get older. We use "fate" to explain many crucial events because evolutionary genes pushed us around against our will so much when we were young. "Fate" thinking is a hard habit to break, but it comes at a time of life where it actually has become breakable, when a change in behavior is possible.

Logical explanations are not the only persuaders, because we all feel in our bones the change that takes place in our lives after 50. We say we mature; we say we get wise. We feel it although we may not act on it. Anyway, it occurs and we sense it to varying degrees.

The problem with such maturing lies in the structure of habit. If we can change a habit, or learn a new habit, we need to first believe we can do it and then we have to reconcile ourselves to the time it takes to break old habits and to acquire new ones.

Habits get ingrained very quickly in us as babies and as young children. In early life habit-learning gets a jump start because all our mental reactions are developing at a fast pace. Some results come from our genes, of course, and some from imitation of peers and elders. But hard-wired reaction or a soft-wired habit, both come easily and fast and automatically in the first few years of life. Not so when we are adults.

In the second half of life when we are in the habit-changeable part, we forget how long it takes to break old habits or to form new ones—far longer than it did in our youth. Both habit and gene behavior look the same. Is change worth it? This possibility-of-change period is difficult and long. Should we persist if we are not sure it will help?

We now know enough to say with confidence that after 50 change can occur and will pay off. Before 50 we can't be so sure change will occur; we may run into gene-determined "stuff" and be doomed to fail. But after age 50, decisions about change will succeed if we persist.

Degeneration Rates

You may be getting bored by my dilating on heredity and habit for so long, but it is basic to my point that we've slipped very suddenly into a bad habit of inactivity in civilized living. And a basic knowledge of genes and habit can get us out of the trouble.

From what we now know about human lifelines there seem to exist two decay pathways that lead to our inevitable deaths: a natural one and a disease one (See Graph 1).

The natural decay of a human life is measured by scientists from the number of cell divisions that a human cell will undergo before entirely dying out (apoptosis). This number seems to be about 40 cell divisions. We can't exactly figure how many years it should take a human, composed of three trillion cells, to die a natural death. We just guess. Our guesses get longer and longer all the time. Experts now estimate people may live to 110-120 years in the next century.

The second decay pathway, the one where chronic diseases hasten natural decay, is measured by the average mortality statistics reported by public health agencies. These numbers get more precise as the years go by. They show we actually now live about 75 years. The difference between the two pathways of decline is now about

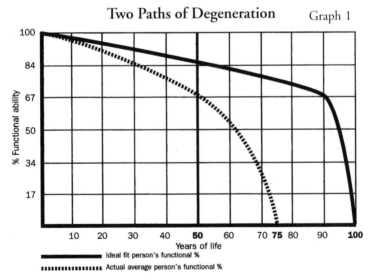

Two Paths of Degeneration   Graph 1

This difference is accounted for by preventable degeneration.

25 years (see Graph 1). The difference narrowed very fast in the early part of the 20th century but is diminishing today at a much slower rate. The reason for this slowing of pace is one subject of this book. That subject, precisely, is this: we have slipped into a civilization-determined habit of sitting still instead of the biologically normal state of standing and moving. This adverse habit can only be corrected by another habit, a new habit which I will soon describe.

The Wellness Triple

Consider the present status of chronic degenerative ailments in our modern society today, which are subject to habit change, and the various measures we are taking to get them under control. Three main population-wide activities aim at increasing wellness: 1) Medical Care; 2) Diet; 3) Exercise.

1. Medical Care

Thousands of books are published each year about the chronic diseases that beset mankind and the means by which modern medicine grapples with them. Now that war, pestilence, accidental deaths and infant mortality are under some control, chronic death-dealers consume increasing amounts of our attention, energy and money. Among these ills are heart disease, cancer, stroke, diabetes, dependency and dementia.

Today we trust the medical care system to care for and control these disorders. But medical care has problems within itself. For one, it struggles under the heel of the business of medical insurance, so that what medical care delivers is warped by huge expense for the patient and huge amounts of time needed to get medicine's benefits. An offshoot of this economic restructuring of American health care is the new custom of many doctors becoming employees, rather than continuing in medicine's tradition as professionals. Two, medical care works under an inherent weakness—it operates by dividing chronic degeneration into 20 or more seperate divisions (diseases) and then devises diagnosis and treatment for each one seperately.

Therefore, patients end up overwhelmed by the multiple pill schedules that constantly change, and multiple sub-specialist visits for multiple diagnostic checks. This activity level is not insignificant; it amounts to half of older-age activity! A major coordination problem exists. Humans do not handle this procedural complexity well, and it gets worse every year.

Big Mother

There is a third difficulty with American medicine that deserves a look. Medical care is more and more coming to assume the role of Big Mother in our lives. George Orwell satirized "Big Brother" as the ultimate force of government in society, taking care of people completely by political dominance. Nowadays we seem to elevate medicine to the role of Big Mother through health care dominance. We love to be taken care of; we love to shift responsibility for our lives; people want a superior force or organization to lead them. Organized medicine seems to qualify for the role by its scientific knowledge, and by its tradition of laying down health rules. Medicine also does the research to establish such authority. America appears to want medicine to fill the Big Mother role.

Who will expose the Big Mother hoax? In the spite of the acknowledged miracles and advances that we all value and need, medicine cannot completely take over the direction of our lives. Medicine is good, but not that good. Each individual is the supreme director of his or her life; medicine can only help and guide. Medicine needs to redirect people's attention to their own inner resources, both physical and mental, so that innate defenses and recovery powers can operate freely and can support the advances of medical care.

No wonder medicine is not rescuing us quicker from premature deaths. It is expensive, piecemeal, and doesn't get to the public as a whole. It will have to develop a public preventive medicine campaign of wide scope if it is to influence the current trend toward inaction and Big Mother dependency and ignorance of how to use innate recovery forces built into our individual constitutions.

One hundred years ago a great doctor named Walter Cannon described the human body's wonderful survivability in possessing "homeostasis"—the strong, built-in power that maintains functional bodily integrity in the face of outside threats such as drought, starvation, injury, etc. Our bodies have inner, automatic recovery mechanisms to keep going on an even keel even when threatened by annihilation. These forces work in us today to keep physiologic integrity in the face of modern threats like inaction, overeating, various drugs and all the other pleasure addictions that modern man uses. My point is that the medical care establishment has not addressed how to keep these inner powers of recovery working well.

I certainly don't imply I know all the answers to this. But I am suggesting a route to begin to help inner health defenses augment the medical care system.

2. Diet

I know in my heart that all the current worry and wrangling over diet is a smokescreen that obscures the basic facts of the failure to control obesity. The facts are unpalatable to many people, and that constitutes part of the problem.

Here's the fact: we all eat too much. There are starving children all over the world about which I feel as sad and guilty as the next person. But in developed countries like America hardly anyone dies of starvation anymore. Those humans in America's past who died of starvation did so for various reasons—food shortage, crop failures, war isolation, ignorance and abject poverty. Today we live in the middle of relative plenty. Today, when someone dies of starvation there is public outrage, because it just shouldn't happen.

But hunger? That is a totally different matter. Hunger is not starvation. Hunger is not really suffering, even though compassionate people cry that no one should "go hungry."

Hunger is the natural feeling built into us to remind us we need food for more energy. Everybody who is not sick feels hunger every morning on awakening. It is our safety response carried over from primitive ages.

Here's the problem, and the irony: today, with food plentiful, we constantly override our hunger signal—or rather the signal that hunger has been satisfied. Today we overeat for all sorts of reasons that can be summed up as "pleasure." The detailed excuses we use are the following: overeating is the only socially acceptable pleasure;

it's a childhood-instilled habit you can't break; it's a failure of parental discipline; it's a peer pressure matter you can't resist; it's the sit-down life that encourages over-eating; it's a school error and teaching failure. Take your pick, or pick all of the above—which one, or all, doesn't make much difference. The discussion always ends with no decision, no solution, no plan for a remedy. Food is our national comfort, a reward for effort, a solace in time of stress, our only completely acceptable addiction.

We all over-eat to a level seldom realized. We all eat at least *twice* the amount we absolutely need for the amount of energy expended in our sit-down existence. We can exist in good health with 1200 calories a day in our sitting society. But average caloric intake runs at least to 2400 calories. Most people eat closer to three times their need. Some eat five times their need.

But why should a "little" excess hurt, since doctors know the human body handles excess? It hurts because the present huge, excessive, over-eating binge by the public is enough to overcome our natural safety factors. People have gone berserk in their overeating for comfort or for relief of stress.

The point about diet in this problem of overeating and illness is that the detailed components of the daily diet pale in importance to the vital overriding fact of eating too much, of eating too many calories. People don't know they eat too much. Expert public discussions on obesity hardly ever mention over-eating! We assume we can eat as much as we want because that's the greatest pleasure in life for most everyone. The current dialogue stands with this satement: "If only we can decide what particular foods are best for us, we will have solved the problem." The real issue of over-eating is lost or ignored. No wonder obesity worsens in the face of all the expert attention. Don't misunderstand—I am not forgetting that we need a balanced diet of carbohydrates, fats and proteins. But the precise proportion of each one doesn't matter as much as *total calories*.

We over-eat these days because we have grown accustomed to the habit of stuffing ourselves to feel full while inactive—not listening to the hunger signal and quitting when hunger is satisfied. Getting the "full" feeling after eating each meal is the path to early death; not death before 50 perhaps, but probably death by 70. Total caloric intake is each person's own individual responsibility, not the job of family, friends, society or the medical profession. Doctors can only urge people to keep their eyes on the main issue.

A reasonable daily caloric intake for adults is about 2,200 calories per day. Most of us average well over 3,000 calories. We can learn to count calories or to measure portions of food. Caloric value booklets abound. However, we need a new standarized unit of food serving; in fact, the word "serving" is too elastic. A "level teaspoon" would be more accurate. Nutritionists can make this decision for a new standard to help people plan better. Weight Watchers, for one, has done this.

How do we face the real issue of overeating, especially when one does it as a main pleasure in life? The public has to experiment with caloric curtailment individually. People first can realize that they "stuff" at meals to get that "full feeling." Then they have to suffer for about two or three weeks with a reduced intake that fails to "fill" them but satisfies hunger. This is the tough period. But if they can suffer through it, they get a new habit; instead of feeling full they feel free of that logy laziness after meals that accompanies stuffing.

The reward for this is weight loss. But you can't rely on weight loss as your only reward. Your new "unstuffed" habit gets its reinforcement from slower eating to enjoy each mouthful thoroughly. Well-prepared, delicious food deserves a calm slowness to appreciate fully its flavor and goodness. This slow pace was the key feature of old-fashioned family meal rituals, which fostered real enjoyment of each dish and eating what you felt you wanted by need, not by greed or by time demand.

To correct our society-wide overeating habit we need to change our thoughts about food. First, we need to eat only the amount of food that satisfies hunger; we must develop ways to dispose of excess food—freeze it, save it, or give it to the homeless; at least throw it out rather than eat it. (Think of the huge amounts of food restaurants throw out. You are cutting your life short if you eat it.)

Each day that you read and hear about obesity and the related illness it causes is a day you realize that arguing about specific food substances, or taking dietary supplements, is not helping. The ailments of over-eating steadily worsen. But we laugh and open another carton of snack food. The majority of us don't know any other way to enjoy life.

A leading expert on obesity was interviewed in a recent issue of the *Journal of the American Medical Association*. Summarizing studies on the treatments and diets for obesity, he concluded that "obesity is a very complex *social* problem as well as a medical problem."

3. Exercise

As we use the word today, exercise is far too diverse and unfocused to affect any concrete, population-wide change of trend. Exercise means 20 different forms of activity to 20 different groups of people. Exercise in general, and each specific form of it in particular, may only be as good as the full breathing and posture recovery it engenders. (I'll explain this later). For now, let's examine what popular versions of exercise actually do for us.

I speak about exercise for two reasons: 1) 1 have spent my life as an enthusiast for various forms of exercise as befitted my age. I did all games and sports as a youngster (school and college competitive sports at high levels); I continued tennis, swimming, running and golf every few days to keep in shape during my active surgery years. I jogged and walked and golfed regularly during my older years. And in between these sports I did "sitting-up exercises" that combined sit-ups, push-ups, pull-ups, head stands, and a few other moves from school and college training sessions. In short, I felt in my gut the results of the common exercises that most other people do and I can compare them with the bodily and mental emotional states I experienced while doing the various ones.

2) 1 have spent my professional and personal life studying the physical reactions of various ages to different life situations and to various disease states. This gives me a perspective that is hard to acquire from books.

All of these various forms of exercise that I did had

disappointing results when considered as candidates for a national program to improve fitness. Organized sports can only be valuable for coordinated, exercise-educated persons who naturally enjoy them. They are generally for the young. They will never attract or be a habit with the majority of people.

Swimming, running and gym workouts depend upon facilities and weather; they are often costly; they are too strenuous for most people; they are intermittent and seemed planned to last for only a few years. All of these versions carry some risk of injury and require doctor's clearances.

Exercise as pursued today in America works to correct the inactivity part of our modern sedentary predicament, and that's fine. But the *sitting* part remains unaddressed. Lifelong sitting distorts a particular segment of our bodies—the lower back—and this requires a particular solution not faced by *general* exercise. There needs to be a solution everybody can use, because everybody sits most all day. My solution is the **Seven Essential Exercises Daily** (I'll refer to this set of exercises as SEED throughout this book). SEED restores the supple, natural back that we all lose from sitting by the time we reach middle age. SEED restores erect, easy movement to enable functioning into old age.

Aerobics addresses one aspect of fitness—endurance. SEED addresses another aspect—lifelong upright functionability.

Walking

Walking is the only exercise that everybody can engage in, can possibly enjoy, can afford, and which carries no risk. The only trouble is that one has to walk a long, long time to get desirable results. There is no feeling of well-being from walking that is noticeable to me as I do it. Also, when I was having back pain attacks connected to golfing, walking never helped. In some ways it qualifies for a national program—it is free for everyone, risk free, and can be done inside on a treadmill when the weather is bad. But it is *so* boring! Even with a Walkman. It's only reward to me is the moral one—you carried out the assigned task, you were faithful to the program. No large clinical, controlled, double-blind study has been inspired by walking. I doubt that national longevity trends would respond to an increase in the walking habit. The best thing about walking is true for any form of activity: some is better than none. That stands as a solid fact. But just telling people to get going and moving doesn't solve the sit-down trap. It is far too inadequate, too general, too much like the cluckings of a mother hen.

Authorities recommend walking one half hour several times a week. That's fine. I often do it and so do millions of others. But the populace as a whole regards this as "good advice to children." It has no gut-appeal; there are no teeth to the recommendation.

Experts on public health realize that more specific exercise recommendations would exclude large segments of the population. For example, sports and workouts exclude the old, yoga excludes the fat, swimming excludes the poor, etc. Where is something specific that works for everyone?

I feel the time is ripe for a new advance. The administration of more medications seems futile. I urge a new, family-instigated, medically-based habit, unified around the idea of correcting for the inaction-sitting trap we have created. Not that some logical thinking isn't needed to create such a correction. But the laissez-faire, hit-or-miss, trial-and-error, muddling-through effort that is the official national policy today is not working. Modern medical care, dietary "advances", and multiple forms of exercise are not getting the job done. Population-wide fitness is becoming worse, not better, as shown by increasing obesity, the rising prevalence of degenerative diseases and early-age disability.

I am not recommending a new habit to replace medical care or diet or general forms of exercise. Just the opposite. I suggest a new medically-based habit added to the established procedures each one of us already tries to use. I don't propose a substitute. I suggest an addition. We need what we already have; we now need to strengthen civilized living.

Mid-Life Profiles

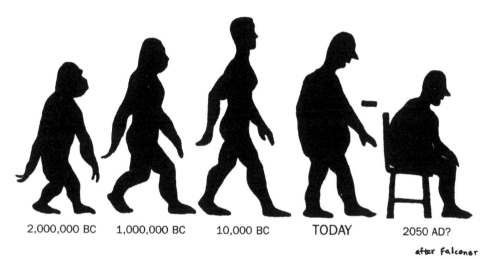

2,000,000 BC   1,000,000 BC   10,000 BC   TODAY   2050 AD?

after falconer

Chapter 3 _____
OUR SITTING EXISTENCE

To recount my experience with back rehabilitation I must tell of some key thoughts that kept occurring to me as I experimented daily for many months with some home floor calisthenics.

The first idea that kept recurring was that humans were made for action. We evolved to survive in the wilderness; that meant heavy active movement of all kinds to get water, food, clothing, shelter and at the same time create families and protect them from predators of all kinds. Humans needed large strong bodies with keen brains to survive in the world that existed many years ago. And survive they did.

The second thought that followed the first was that only in the last 5000 years, a drop in the evolutionary time bucket, has civilization developed in more than half of the human world. This civilization is so recent but so completely transforming. Today it brings us a conquered environment, plenty of food, water, clothing, shelter and hardly any threats from predators compared to caveman days. So our bodies, made for action, now suddenly find no use for the strength and the mobility that preserved us through the ages.

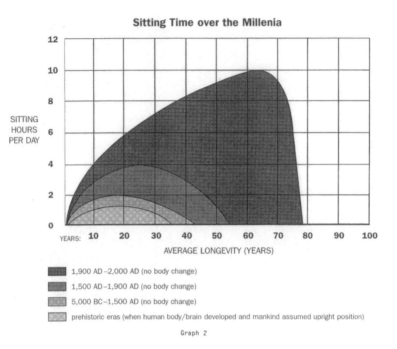

Sitting Time over the Millenia

SITTING HOURS PER DAY

YEARS:

AVERAGE LONGEVITY (YEARS)

■ 1,900 AD –2,000 AD (no body change)
■ 1,500 AD –1,900 AD (no body change)
■ 5,000 BC –1,500 AD (no body change)
▢ prehistoric eras (when human body/brain developed and mankind assumed upright position)

Graph 2

Third, I began to think of civilized living today in more detailed terms of activity. I realized humans now have substituted sitting down for the action-packed daily existence they were made for. We've comparatively stopped moving. We sit most of our waking hours in seats travelling, at desks gazing at screens, in chairs gazing at screens, in seats at theaters and arenas.

No doubt exists that in the last 50 years our society has changed radically as a result of automobiles and television. American industrial capacity has produced cars, trucks, buses, and highways in great profusion. Television sets have become so common that no family or adult is without one, almost regardless of how much a person can afford. The poor, the homeless in shelters, the vagrants in temporary quarters or cared for by agencies, the indigent in public housing or nursing homes--even they all have television. These people aren't out in the cold walking, moving. There is scarcely a significant amount of the population considered rural any more. Farmers need second jobs to survive; they travel in cars. You can't sell or even give away old T.V. sets. Everyone has found a way and a place to sit for events, play, leisure, any type of existence, just in the last 50 or so years. We are already seeing the effects of this massive shift in civilized behavior to sitting and inactivity. We've become a society of obese people.

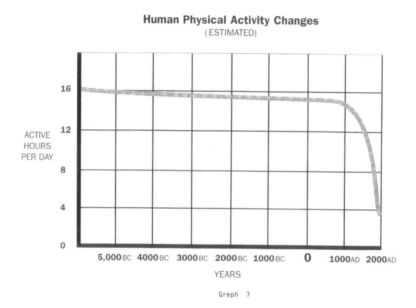

Graph 3

Finally, I put these ideas together with my back problem and got the picture. No wonder my back hurt. I had distorted it by sitting for a lifetime, like everybody else does. My back was made for standing and moving with a necessary double-S spine curve, not for sitting still with a C-curve (see Figure 2.)

Even though I personally stood to operate a few hours a day when performing surgery, I essentially was inactive in order to concentrate 10 of 16 working hours. Most people today remain basically motionless in sitting down 12 to 14 hours a day.

31

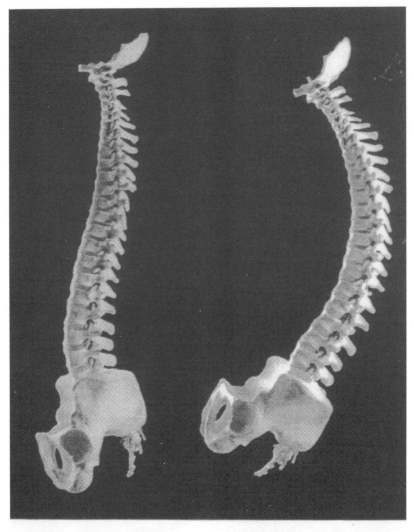

Standing Spine   Sitting Spine
Figure 2.

And what does this lifetime structural distortion do? It "rusts" and stiffens joints, weakens muscles; joints then hurt to move and muscles tear easily with sudden movement.

I was beginning to see why the simple home exercises I was testing made me feel better and reduced my back aches. I began to see why everybody had back pains. I began to see why health authorities just recommended "any exercise at all" that suited people—any movement helped a little. I began to see why individuals embrace such varied exercise routines—any movement was of some help to correct for sitting. But this was so unfocused. My trouble was in my low back, in the lumbar vertebral joints 4 and 5, and in the lumbar-sacral area. That was where my friends felt pain too.

The more I pondered while doing the full-breathing with calisthenics, the more convinced I became that focused correction of the lifelong distortion of the lower back would bring the quickest relief to the weak point of civilized living and possibly begin a cascade of recoveries to other bodily processes that suffer decline as we age.

I now began to realize that if people were to survive well today in the sitting, inactive cyber-age that is now in place, they would need a widespread, daily, new correction habit that was standardized, tested and targeted at the focal point of the sitting trouble.

Chapter 4 ————————————————
HOW SITTING HURTS US

Before I explore the back mobility-breathing-exercise habit that I have settled on, I need to elaborate further on the downside of a sitting life.

Today we work and reproduce and raise families mostly while sitting, not while standing, walking or running. We can think better, get information quicker, communicate easier, travel further and faster when sitting than when standing or walking. But standing upright and moving is what we are biologically structured to do. All of our body functions (therefore brain and mental function as well) are designed for the erect, moving state, not the crouched-over, sitting-still position. Yet in the technical modern world we can't stand or walk or otherwise move a lot and compete. In this cyberage the more we sit, the stiller we keep ourselves concentrating intensely on the road ahead, the television screen or the stage or arena, the more successful lives we lead.

Civilized society doesn't know about the downside of sitting. Sitting embodies the best example of what's bad about too much of a good thing. Mae West said "too much of a good thing is wonderful." She was talking about sex. Sitting is not sex. Today we are overdoing sitting in spades but we don't know it. It's not wonderful. It may be necessary, but has its bad side.

What we haven't yet grasped is that constant sitting over a lifetime deforms our bodies past recall. It disturbs our balance in walking, reduces all joint flexibility (not just the back), dries and "rusts" joints, shallows breathing, slows circulation, slows digestion, slow secretion and waste disposal processes, probably impairs immune response and generally hastens our degeneration rate. (Figure 3.)

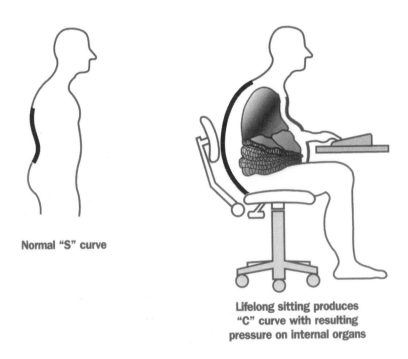

Normal "S" curve

Lifelong sitting produces
"C" curve with resulting
pressure on internal organs

Figure 3.

How can anything as restful as sitting inflict all that harm? Easily. By beginning in early childhood, increasing through all stages of schooling, becoming mandatory in the work-place seven hours a day. By our habit of always traveling in vehicles, and by sitting all day in retirement, sitting down becomes our whole existence. All told, it now encompasses 80-90% of modern waking life.

If our bodies (and this means brains also) were designed for a sit-down life, we could live for 100 years in painless comfort with our present lifestyle. But we were made for action. Action while awake and upright keeps our reparative and defensive machinery working well. In the primitive world action normally occupied two-thirds of the day, and sleep occupied one-third. That was life's program during most of evolving human time. No more.

How Much Do We Sit?

We now sit 80% of our waking hours—at least 12 of every 15 hours out of bed. There is no period of life when sitting does not dominate. Published medical authorities all agree with this figure. I measured my own sitting time during an ordinary day. It came to just over 12 hours in a 15-hour day. (I have spent about 9 hours a day in bed since I reached the age of 70).

Hundreds of persons have talked to me about sitting. They ranged from 45 to 75 years of age, both men and women, from all strata of society, with a wide assortment of occupations. Their average sitting time comes out much the same as mine. Some eat out and sit longer; many go to movies, shows, sports arenas and sit longer. While it varies some, everybody sits most of the time (Graph 3).

Younger adults may sit less than this because child-rearing is more motion-packed. Our car culture increases yearly the time spent sitting and travelling to ever farther-removed places. Younger people may engage in active sports. However, older folks sit all day long every day. "Rockin' chair's got me" fits most of the elderly; (the newer chair designs now make the rocking chair obsolete.) Elderly backs are so stiff in the distorted, bent forward position (see Fig. 3) that a chair is their natural habitat. Getting up from the chair is a strain and a pain and sometimes a danger; the sudden instability may cause a fall and a broken bone.

Half of activity for an older person nowadays is getting up from sitting and sitting back down. The gods of our forefathers

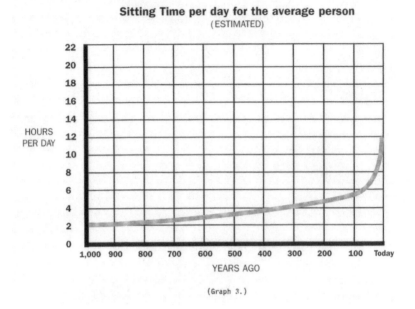

Sitting Time per day for the average person
(ESTIMATED)

(Graph 3.)

must be crying out seeing our miraculous bodies being so wasted.

The conclusion from such a sedentary review is that sitting all day is all-pervasive; it increases rapidly each year as civilized gadgets make life easier; it is seldom considered harmful, only restful; and it is absolutely necessary to our living a modern life.

Specific Ailments From Sitting

When I say that ailments come from sitting, I don't mean that I have proved this experimentally in a laboratory. Biology students in the future may devise tests and see abnormalities develop that don't occur in ambulatory controls. I'm relying on my well-tested powers of observation, common sense and on my professionally disciplined habit of accuracy (60 research publications). Another bit of evidence: most people I have talked with over the years agree that these conclusions accord with common knowledge.

Three Classes of Ailments

Three classes of ailments are related to lifelong sitting down: 1) Low back pain; 2) a hindering of specific vital functions-like breathing and circulation; 3) chronic diseases that progress quicker from mild to severe with inactivity.

1. Back Pain

Many sources of back pain exist. The most common is mechanical in nature, not from injury. It is a chronic, low back hurting that occurs with ordinary movement, such as bending, lifting, getting up, sitting down or walking.

The sitting position flattens the normal anterior curve of the lower spine, albeit a mild normal curve (as shown on page 36) which was put there to support efficiently the main weight of the body when standing and walking or running. Sitting changes this curve, tends to bow it backwards and fix it in an abnormal curve tending to a backward reverse curve, that makes us look somewhat stooped over. Most people over 55 therefore stand and walk awkwardly, bent forward, off balance, uncertain of gait, weight unevenly distributed on legs and feet because their lower back becomes fixed in this abnormal position. This backward-bent lower back constitutes the point of back troubles. It is the key angle of back positioning; it is the heart of the sitting problem.

We have 100 separate joints in our spines, half of all the joints in the body. They are not very apparent because they only move through small ranges of motion. But they wouldn't be present for millions of years unless they were vital. They enable motion in the erect position and facilitate breathing adequately while moving and walking, etc. The whole spinal framework is wonderfully engineered to perform vital functions while erect and moving. Low back joints are crucial to this plan. Sitting all our lives constitutes inaction which leads to stagnation of functions, but also imposes joint fusing, "rusting", drying, thinning of joint spaces, and "spurring" (calcium deposits), and consequent low back pain on attempts to stand and move. All of us have observed the spontaneous fusion of a joint from prolonged disuse—an arm in a sling for two months may never rise normally again.

Normal alignment of our lower back gets so fixed in an awkward position from sitting that in middle age we all succumb to it. We know our bodies are stiff and hurt but the natural urge to stretch and bend to return to nature's planned moving position gives only more pain so we quit that, and accept the disability. This disability solidifies more and the trouble builds faster and faster; the more we sit, the more we have to sit. To be good optimistic citizens and set our children and grandchildren a good example, we accept our fate and smile. It is really a lousy example to set for future life.

The corollary ailment to low back pain from awkward lower spine stiffening is easy injury from ordinary activities. A stiff spine is an injury waiting to happen. Lifelong sitting fixes the spine in a poor weight-bearing alignment; muscles and ligaments are already weak from years of inaction and they are therefore not of a size or shape to support a mal-aligned pile of spinal bones. Thus when a middle-aged person has to make some quick, coordinated movement like bending, twisting, or lifting, their back "goes out." Severe pain ensues; visits to doctors, x-rays, perhaps myelograms follow. They always show up some defect that years of sitting has caused. Many such persons end up with a spine operation for a "slipped disc," a narrowed space pressing on a nerve or other anatomical flaw. Then more enforced rest weakens all structures further and yields a permanently "bad" back that ensures disability for life.

Keeping a supple lower back develops a habit of good anatomical position and can forestall the above story. Just sitting still in good position is not the answer, either. Chairs that help good sedentary posture may help a little; but they don't solve the back pain problem.

2. Stagnation of Vital Functions

Breathing bears the brunt of sitting-down constriction of function. Forward crunching while sitting compresses the lungs inside the rib cage, pushes down on the abdominal organs below and compresses them (stomach, intestines, liver, and large veins carrying blood back to the heart for reoxygenation). (See Figure 4.) This hampers the main breathing muscle, the diaphragm, that descends normally to expand the lungs. The diaphragm is a thin sheet of muscle that is easily interfered with by this increased abdominal pressure. The resulting smaller volume of air-exchange gets to be a habit after years of sitting forward in rapt concentration.

Finally the hard-wired breathing reflex that keeps us alive adapts at a lower level and we breathe far shallower in mid-life than serves optimal functioning of mind and body. In later life we have to make an effort to breathe fully and deeply. Our respiratory mechanism has shifted from serving action to serving inaction and we begin to feel half dead. (See also later Chapter on Breathing).7

On top of breathing constriction, sitting crunched forward all our lives compresses our internal mid-body organs. Circulation of blood and lymph to essential organs get slowed. The large veins that return blood to the heart for more oxygen get easily compressed. Other digestive and immune resonses and waste disposal mechanisms also slow down.

Such depression of vital processes can be withstood by young persons pretty well because of the vigorous recovery powers of healthy bodies and the excess capacity nature provides. But after the age of

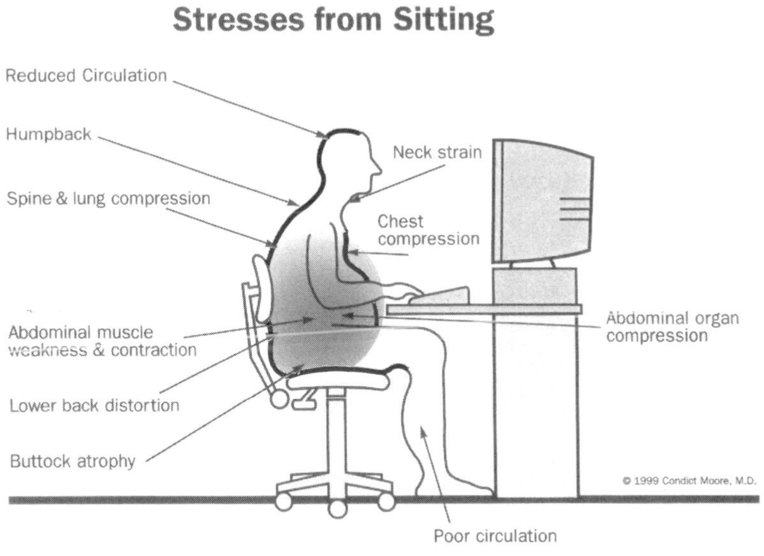

Stresses from Sitting

Reduced Circulation

Humpback

Spine & lung compression

Neck strain

Chest compression

Abdominal muscle weakness & contraction

Abdominal organ compression

Lower back distortion

Buttock atrophy

Poor circulation

© 1999 Condict Moore, M.D.

Figure 4.

50 we begin to use up our reserves; recovery falters. And the more we sit, the quicker we age, unless we learn to correct for it.

Waste disposal comprises another vital body function that is affected. If unneeded substances in food, water and air are not processed by our bodies and excreted efficiently they will accumulate in our tissues in various forms (plaques in blood vessels, fat in all soft parts and organs, calcium in joints, "fibrillary tangles" in and around brain cells*). These accumulations form the basis of many degenerative diseases; slowing of excretion mechanisims can hasten the progress of these diseases. We can easily imagine that prolonged inaction in our lives slows excretory activity and quickens waste accumulation in various parts in organs.

3. Chronic Disability

Medicine began studying aging only recently; it doesn't give any attention as yet to the role of overwhelming inactivity on lives that were made for activity. The basic change-over in human lifestyle occurred too recently to sink into popular awareness. We weren't made to be mental beings totally; we've got to face this and adjust. Life is in one sense a race with death. The only way we can win is to postpone death; we can't escape it. The decay process that leads inevitably to our death begins in early adult life and then it gathers steam and speeds up a lot in older age.

Medical science is just beginning to learn about the essentials of the degeneration rate in humans. The slow aging of normal cells is a process that takes many years. We are studying more and more intensely the degenerative diseases that hasten this normal decay. These diseases are heart disease, cancer, stroke, arthritis, diabetes, demmentia, obesity, etc. If those conditions begin early in the course of our lives, they kill us off quite soon unless controlled. If these decay conditions occur in later middle-age they progress at a faster rate in some persons than in others; those people then die sooner than need be. The degenerative diseases cut life shorter than normal

---

*Authorities don't agree that the fibrillary tangles in the brain of Alzheimer's patients is from poor waste disposal but that is a leading hypothesis.

cell deterioration. That is all pretty obvious. The point is that the time of onset and rate of progression of these degenerations can be controlled; they are not inevitable fixed-rate afflictions visited upon us by nature, independent of our control.

Humans can put up with a gradual decay process that creeps upon us slowly enough so we can accomodate to the slowing of functioning without feeling depressed. It is the "quicker-than-normal" pace of decay that we instinctively feel is unfair and depresses us because we believe deep down that it would have been different and better if we'd been more aware.

These ideas have been constantly in my own mind as I have watched the decay, both normal and disease caused, progress in my own life since the age of 65. 1 have had severe injuries from falls, reparative operations, chronic lung disease and infection from years of younger age smoking, heart rate disturbances, prostatism but no cancer yet, optical cataracts and deafness and memory slowness. I've had it all but cancer and stroke and early dementia. Most of what I've had has been treated. I'll have the last three certainly if I live long enough.

My degeneration rate, seemingly average in my 70's, has slowed in my 80's. My attrition rate must be fairly normal but the degenerative disease attrition rate seems to have slowed down. In fact, I feel so much better in my 80's than I did in my 70's that I feel revived. Of course I move more slowly now and cannot perform vigorous functions.

But I can still function by working in an office every day, studying, playing golf, writing, communicating, using my particular experience productively.

The important thing to me is that I am not disabled. Most of my contemporaries are either dead or disabled. Warding off disability from the degenerative diseases thus becomes the job of later life. From my experience with it so far I firmly believe it is a controllable, manageable part of aging. It will respond to analysis and planning. SEED is the beginning of that plan to delay degenerative disease progression.

The rate of progression of degenerative diseases like heart

disease, cancer and stroke, etc. is not a fixed rate but a variable one. This rate can be slowed so we live to be 100 or thereabouts. Sixty thousand Americans have done it. Authoritives believe 110 to 120 will be achieved ages in the next few generations. Increasing inactivity speeds up the rate; daily corrective conditioning slows it down. The rest of this book describes the simple correction I am talking about. I haven't proved in the laboratory that inactivity pure and simple speeds up degenerative disease progression but I have done the opposite: I've experimentally showed that activity slows overt cancer appearance in animals. Cancer is now explained as a time-dependent accumulation of special mutations of cells. If this accumulation rate responds to activity differences, then other degenerative conditions could be expected also to so respond.Suffice it to say I have formed a conviction that gets stronger each year: degeneration of our lives as measured by the rate of advancement of degenerative diseases can be slowed by concentrating on the daily correction of sitting distortion of our bodies. Disability can be delayed in this way by an average of 20 years and enjoyable life prolonged.

I will have more to say about where inactivity-correction fits into modern medical care.

Chapter 5 _____
SOLVING THE SITTING PROBLEM

Sitting needs to be broken down into several components if it is to be solved as a problem. There are three parts:

1) General inactivity. Sitting involves being physically still. Most people get at the immobility of modern life through general exercise programs like sports, gym workouts, yoga, walking, running, etc. Such activity constitutes a fairly good solution to general immobility but not for the other components.

2) Posture distortion. This part of the sitting problem gets some attention and a halfway solution by ergonomics. Chair design and planning for a good sitting position has advanced so that intelligent planning is possible to enable all sitters to achieve good lower back repositioning. But static repositioning restores only at most half of what we lose in a life of sitting. Ergonomics helps keep good posture and helps prevent back ache but it does not recover function and mobility.

3) Back fixation and loss of suppleness. Here is the component that exercise specialists and chair designers have forgotten. It is the fixation and stiffness in an off-balanced alignment that prevents good function and creates pain on even moderate movement. This stiffness arises from lack of motion of the lower back joints. The awkward stiffness makes a natural, balanced, erect posture an effort and a chore.

I visualize the unsolved sitting problem as mainly a joint problem, with muscle weakness second in importance. If any human joint is kept still and unmoving for two months or more, it may never regain full motion. Such is the natural scenario of joint physiology. Joints need fluid—tiny amounts to be sure—but real fluid nonetheless, to move easily and painlessly. Fluid must get into a joint space between and around the bony-cartilaginous surfaces that rub over one another; it gets there by the pumping action of joint motion. We must move our joints to keep them in lubricated shape. An unmoving joint quickly becomes stiff and dry. Also, still joints accumulate waste materials, like calcium deposits, that limit range of motion. When motion returns to a joint, pain is induced, which engenders more immobility to avoid pain. The process then snowballs. Joint dysfunction becomes arthritis which leads eventually to total disability.

This sequence omits mentioning the muscle weakness that accompanies joint immobility; weak muscles tear easier on ordinary movement. And remember, the back has half of the joints of the whole body. The joints were put there to move, not fuse into solid rods.

When my back pain was the worst I was given the diagnosis of "facetitis" by my neurosurgeon. That meant that the tiny bony projections on either side of each vertebral body were inflamed and irritated. The main back joints, the intervertebral spaces, have cushions (discs). But the facets are regular joints. They often account for low back pain.

Unless we face this loss of flexibility of the lower back, we cannot expect to reverse the inactivity-sitting-damage trend now engulfing us. The good news is this: the bad effects of lifelong sitting can be reversed by the Seven Essential Exercises Daily habit I describe in the following pages. Remember, trend reversal requires more than general activity; it needs a highly specific, lower back attention every day.

Chapter 6 ——————————————————————
THE SEVEN ESSENTIAL EXERCISES DAILY; THE "SEED" PROGRAM

In the following pages I describe and illustrate the essential exercises, which I call the Seven Essential Exercises Daily, or the SEED program. I add three additional ones that are less essential, but I often do them for posture and balance.

While these moves with deep respiration are the same ones many of us were taught as children by our second grade teachers in public school 80 years ago, they have now acquired a totally new importance and urgency because of the way civilization has developed.

Exercise 1

"Pecs" and "Lats" muscle stretch for back bones adjustment, posture and deep breathing

Time: 11/2 minutes

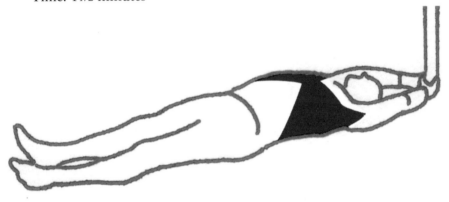

This is a good exercise to begin with. It stretches the entire body, but mainly the anterior and lateral large chest muscles. It expands the chest cavity.

Flatten back against the floor. Place your body so your arms become straight over your head, touching your ears on either side. Grasp a table leg or other heavy object and hold steady for 11/2 minutes, or until the stretching feeling eases.

This position should flatten the lower spine curve as you touch the floor with the entire spine. It loosens the shoulder joints, which lock and stiffen quickly when not put through full range of movement. During this stretch, take 15 slow, very deep breaths.

EXERCISE 1 COMMENTS

The act of flattening all the curves of the spine, from neck to pelvis, on the floor begins the process of unstiffening the spinal joints that sitting has rigidified. It also begins the important lower lumbar curve correction from a forward C-curve to a normal S-curve. You not only begin an easy movement back to nature's proper positioning, you begin restoring normal joint motion and attendant muscle conditioning. This all begins to restore normal posture when you stand.

The act of stretching your arms high above your head by holding on to the legs of some piece of furniture pulls and stretches the "lats" muscles that help expand the chest. This ensures full lung filling and emptying, so that lungs get exercise as well as muscles. The most distant air cells become filled and emptied and the full lung capacity gets used and kept in working order.

To accomplish these several purposes you want to take your time; take at least 12 full breaths without forced breathing or hurrying. These breaths serve to time the exercise.

Exercise 2

Buttock Muscle Strength, for Posture

Time: 1 minute

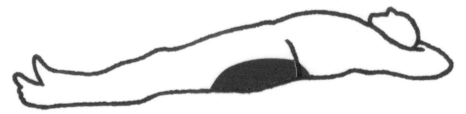

Keep elbows on the floor.

Buttocks muscle strength and tone is crucial to balance; it also strengthens the back wonderfully and prevents back pain. Buttocks are thinned out and are abused continually in sitting. They are the most neglected muscles in the body, also the largest ones.

Flatten your entire back against the floor. You must squeeze (contract) these large muscles strongly, like a pelvic thrust, for a slow count of seven—three as you inhale, then four as you exhale. Repeat ten times.

EXERCISE 2 COMMENTS

You accomplish two objectives with this No. 2 exercise. You restore tone and strength to the largest muscles that control the lower back curve, so critical to a healthy posture. As a case in point, recall the large protruding buttock muscles of healthy young athletes who stand so erectly. The buttock muscles are well and strong and give an unconscious balanced stance to the upright posture. Good buttocks are not all fat.

Secondly, you continue the back suppling and flattening started in Exercise No. 1 by keeping your hands behind your head with elbows touching the floor.

You time the buttock contractions by counting 1 and 2 and 3 and 4 and 5 and 6 for each contraction so that you take six seconds for each one. Breathe slowly and deeply in for 1 and 2, then out fully for 3 and 4 and 5 and 6. Rest on 7, then begin the next contraction.

Exercise 3

"ABS" (Abdominals) Muscle Strength

Time: 45 seconds

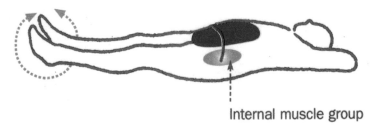

Internal muscle group

Keep elbows touching floor as shown.

This exercise strengthens the "abs", especially the internal muscles that connect to the deep lower back.

Flatten your back against the floor. Raise heels six inches off the floor and circle one foot clockwise, the other counterclockwise 20 times without touching the floor. Then rest. Reverse the movement 20 times the opposite way. Breathe fully during this exercise. Feel the strain deeply in your lower back.

EXERCISE 3 COMMENTS

Physiotherapists often say that the most important muscles for back conditioning are the abdominals. Quite true. This single toning-up and strengthening routine gets at the "stomach" muscles but also strengthens the ilio-psoas muscles deep behind your intestines that help flex your thighs. They pull forward the lumbar spine into normal, anterior curvature.

Many people say this exercise hurts them "deep down inside." That is exactly where you are supposed to feel the pull. If it hurts, it means the important ilio-psoas muscles are too weak and need the strengthening even more than if you felt no strain. Do them in segments if necessary. Don't omit them ever.

Women who have borne babies to term have stretched and weakened all their abdominals to a serious extent. In my experience very few mothers have ever had enough rehabilitation of these muscles to get back to normal for good, natural posture. Doing this exercise, and Exercise No. 4, begins such rehabilitation so necessary to preventing back pain and returning good posture and balance.

Add a leg flutter
- Raise legs in a straight line together.
All hold kicks.
Do not let back arch

Exercise 4 (sit-up)

For "ABS" strengthening; back strengthening and stretching, deep breathing

Time: 1 1/2 minutes

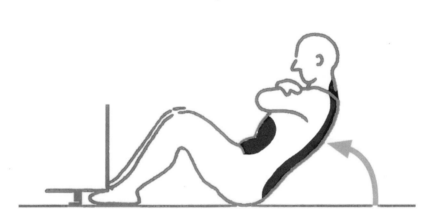

Bend your knees. Place your feet under a sturdy object, such as a sofa, to use feet as a lever. Raise your upper body off the floor with arms crossed on chest.

Sit up as far as possible eight times; count to 3 between sit-ups. Move slowly, evenly, avoid jerky movements. Breathe out fully before each rising; this will tend to flatten your belly, raising your diaphragm more into your chest and allows some displacement of internal organs out of lower abdomen so motion of forward bending is easier.

This movement provides more strenuous exercise than previous ones, gives abdominal strength and mobility to spine joints.

EXERCISE 4 (SIT-UP) COMMENTS

Many people say they can't do this exercise. No need to omit it however; it helps more in the long run if it is difficult at first. Here are several ways to make it easier:

1) Bend knees even more than at right angles, over 90 degrees; this helps leverage.

2) Pad toes so furniture edge doesn't hurt your feet. You depend on your feet to pull hard at first to get the sit-up started.

Place a small towel or washcloth over toes and only insert the toes under the edge of the furniture, not the whole foot. Wear slippers or sport shoes.

3) Forcibly exhale before exerting to begin each sit-up. This flushes air out of the most "far removed" air sacs in the lungs, gives them a good air exchange not usual with ordinary activity. It also reduces the bulk of your belly, which is what gets in the way and obstructs sitting up. It is this belly-bulk that compels most of us to say at the start that we can't do it. Exhaling fully displaces this belly-bulk upwards.

4) Cross hands over chest as shown; this puts your elbows and upper arms in place to lend a weight to lead the first quick burst of effort to sit up. Also push your head forward to help this first burst of effort. You don't need to sit fully vertical to complete each sit-up. I barely touch my elbows to my thighs and then quickly lie back each time. If you can only get your back off the floor at first, the muscle contracture and spine-bending are of benefit. Just persist. You'll get better each day.

Exercise 4A (Alternative Sit-up)

For "abs" strengthening; back strengthening and stretching, deep breathing

Time: 1 1/2 minutes

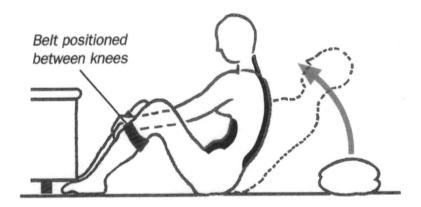

Belt positioned between knees

Women who have borne children often have atrophic, weak abdominal muscles such that they can't easily do the Exercise 4 sit-up. I suggest they sit up as far as they can for 8 tries. Partial sitting up can be done with the "belt technique" shown below. Do this 8 times. Thinned-out muscles will gain strength and their range of motion will improve. Mothers need this strengthening more than other people.

Belt technique: A belt can be placed around both knees, which are spaced a foot apart. Hold the belt with both hands to help raise and lower your body to perform the exercise.

EXERCISE 4A COMMENTS

This alternative belt technique is an interim, half-way method for overweight mothers to begin sit-ups. It uses hands and arms to get over that hurdle of the first rise off the floor. That's where people hurt at the start. The belt technique helps get over the early exertion that discourages people whose abdominals have gotten so weak as to presage early disability as life unfolds. Some persons merely grab the outside of their knees to begin the sit-up.

Start by reaching to knees, lifting
only head, shoulders + upper back

Exercise 5

For spine mobility

Time: 1 minute

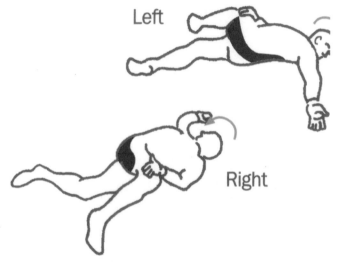

'o not do this exercise if you have had a hip replacement operation.

Here the spinal joints are put through their turning arcs. This stretches all the back-twisting muscles. It also stretches pectorals, neck muscles, and buttocks. It may act like a home chiropractic treatment for spinal bones.

Hold the opposite thigh with the hand, outstretch the other arm and turn the head sharply to the side of the outstretched arm. Hold the position for 10 deep breaths, then switch to the other side for the same. Take time to turn fully and feel the stretch.

This exercise does wonders for your ability to turn your head to see other cars when you are driving. (I feel my neck bones click and pop a little when I do this.)

EXERCISE 5 COMMENTS

One of the most disabling fixations of older age is the inability to turn your head enough to do ordinary living tasks. When your neck gets rigid you can't see objects around you; you fail to see cars at the sides on the road when driving; in general you behave like a disabled oldster who needs someone to care for him or her.

If you are older when you begin this exercise, remember you can restore mobility in spinal turning if you proceed slowly and persistently. Push to twist as far as you can with these two twists and feel the pull on neck and thighs; hold on each side for ten slow, deep breathings in and out.

Don't be alarmed if your spinal bones "click"; that shows you are doing it properly. Of course, don't force this twisting too far to cause permanent pain.

Hip replacement patients may dislocate the artificial joint, especially in the immediate post-operative period, *so they must avoid this exercise.*

Exercise 6

Back Muscle Strengthening

Time: 1 minute

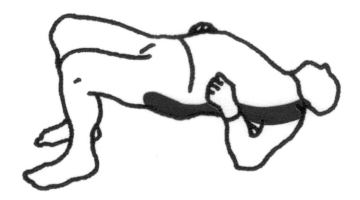

If difficult at first, repeat only 3 times and work up to the recommended 5 times.

This is the best single back conditioner of all.

Lie flat. Bend knees fully and plant feet on floor with heels close to buttocks as possible. Rest elbows on the floor. Push on elbows to raise buttocks and back and shoulders off the floor. You will rest only on feet, elbows and back of head.

Hold for a slow count of 5. Repeat 5 times. You will feel real tension in the neck and at lower curve of the spine, just where you need strength.

Evolution developed these large muscle masses, running up and down along the spine, to hold humans upright. Modern civilized sitting posture entirely neglects them. They get small and weak over the years, allowing sudden movements to cause minor injury.

If difficult at first, repeat only 3 times and work up to the recommended 5 times.

EXERCISE 6 COMMENTS

The key to raising your entire back off the floor is in pushing with your elbows. This places some load and strain on your neck, so be careful here. Don't do the exercise with improper form which causes real pain. You're not supposed to rest your whole body weight directly on the neck. There is some strain on the neck, though, and after a few weeks you will tolerate this. You *need* the strengthening of neck muscles.

This exercise not only strengthens para-spinal muscles that get weak with constant sitting, it also moves your spinal joints to keep them oiled, supple, friction-free and painless.

Arms straight a floor =
glute bridge
ok to stop at shoulders

Exercise 7

Mobility of Neck and Back Joints

Time: 4 minutes

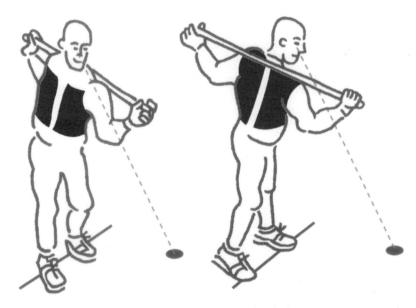

This exercise is most important for balance, posture and golf swing consistency.

Bend knees 10 degrees. Stand upright. Place stick across top of shoulders as shown. Bow from the waist to a comfortable balanced stance—perhaps 10 degrees. Feel solidly balanced. Fix your eyes on a spot 24 inches or so from your feet. Turn slowly and evenly to a comfortable limit to the right until the left shoulder is under the chin, or as near as possible. Keep your eye on the spot and keep feeling perfect balance. Turn back to the left using the same motion taking care not to lean forward. Repeat 35 times. Do it in repetitions of 10 turns at first, with rests between each set of 10.

Remember to breathe fully while doing the slow turns. Turn to the limit each time. You will find that your range of movement increases remarkably as you proceed.

EXERCISE 7 COMMENTS

This is the only exercise done off the floor. It restores and improves standing and balance; it uses spinal joint twisting to keep the 100 or so spinal joint surfaces in smooth working order. If you feel any "clicking" in your spine, it's normal and healthy and needed. Of all the exercises, this one helps most to avoid awkward weight distribution when upright and when walking. You have to assume good spinal positioning to keep doing these 35 times to the right and to the left.

The main cause of older age disability, as I stress often, is poor posture in standing and walking. The spine is curved out of natural alignment so body weight gets shifted forward, requiring constant unnatural effort to stay erect. In this exercise you bend forward very slightly from the hips, compensating by slight knee flexion so your weight gets balanced on your legs without extra effort. Then the turning action reinforces this good, less forward-curved, balanced spine position. When you finish you feel as though you've learned to stand properly again.

As an incidental result, this exercise mimics the basic turn of the golf swing. Keeping perfect balance without moving the head but turning shoulders right and left as fully as possible constitutes the fundamental move of hitting a golf ball percisely. One needs to hit it precisely, accurately, time after time, to make a good score. Nothing I have ever learned or practiced in golf has helped reduce my handicap more than this daily exercise.

I want to devote a small separate chapter to the great value of this exercise to all golfers. Here's where the fun begins. If you don't play golf, you'll have to be content with the postural freedom and exhilaration that Exercise 7 affords.

Optional Leg Muscle Stretches

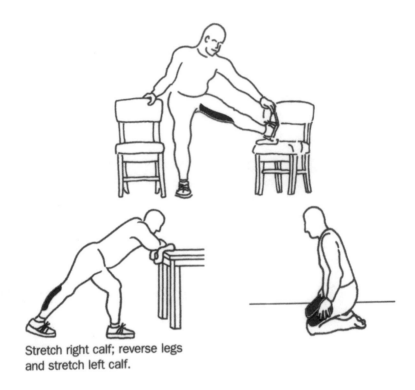

Stretch right calf; reverse legs
and stretch left calf.

These are supplemental and optional to the Seven Essential Exercises Daily (SEED). These leg-stretching exercises help balance and walking, indirectly helping the back. (I do them because they fit easily into my routine)

Do these exercises in whatever sequence you choose. The order is not important; the order here just follows my own personal order of 1 through 7. I have done them in several different sequences and find no virtue in one order over another.

If you do them twice a day you'll get benefits twice as fast to start and feel even better.

Summary Sheet

Seven Essential Exercises Daily (SEED)

(tear out sheet for easy reference)

1. "PECS" & "LATS" STRETCH

Flatten back against the floor. Stretch shoulders and arms so that upper arms touch ears. Breathe deeply 10 times. **Hold steady for 1 1/2 minutes.**

2. BUTTOCK STRENGTHENING

Flatten back against floor. Squeeze (contract) buttocks strongly for a **slow count of 7, 3 as you inhale then relax for a count of 4, repeat 10 times with deep breath each time.**

3. "ABS" (ABDOMINALS) STRENGTHENING

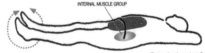

INTERNAL MUSCLE GROUP

Flatten back against floor. Raise heels 6" off the floor. Circle one foot clockwise, the other counterclockwise **20 times** without touching the floor. Rest; repeat in reverse circles. Remember to breathe fully during the "circles".

4. SPINAL MOBILITY

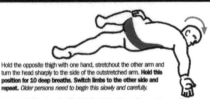

Hold the opposite thigh with one hand, stretch out the other arm and turn the head sharply to the side of the outstretched arm. **Hold this position for 10 deep breaths. Switch limbs to the other side and repeat.** *Older persons need to begin this slowly and carefully.*

Do not do this exercise if you have had a hip replacement operation.

5. BACK MUSCLE STRENGTHENING

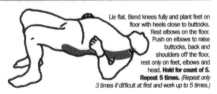

Lie flat. Bend knees fully and plant feet on floor with heels close to buttocks. Rest elbows on the floor. Push on elbows to raise buttocks, back and shoulders off the floor, rest only on feet, elbows and head. **Hold for count of 5. Repeat 5 times.** *(Repeat only 3 times if difficult at first and work up to 5 times.)*

6. "ABS" (ABDOMINALS) STRENGTHENING

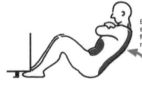

Bend knees. Place feet under sturdy object, such as a sofa, for leverage. After fully exhaling, raise upper body off floor with arms crossed on chest. **Repeat 8 times.**

7. MOBILITY OF NECK AND BACK JOINTS

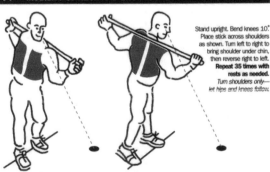

Stand upright. Bend knees 10°. Place stick across shoulders as shown. Turn left to right to bring shoulder under chin, then reverse right to left. **Repeat 35 times with rests as needed.** Turn shoulders only— let hips and knees follow.

© 2003 Condict Moore, M.D.

(Also see Travel Card)

TABLE I

The Seven Exercises That Keep 104 Joints Flexible and Pain Free
(free of painful aftermath from normal activity)

Joints	Exercise Numbers
Shoulders (4)	1,4,5,6,7
Intervertebral joints - neck (21)	5,6,7
thorax (60)	1,5
lumbar (lower back) (15)	2,5,6,7
Hips (4)	2,4,5

The lumbar area joints (lower back where our backs usually hurt from over-sitting) are the important ones that get mobilized. But all spinal joints gain flexibility so I list them all.

TABLE II

The Seven Exercises Condition More Than 50 Muscles

Larger Back Muscles	Numbered exercises that strenghten or stretch particular muscles.
Splenics (neck) (4)	5, 6
Trapezius	6, 7
Sternomastoid	5, 6, 7
Levator scapulae	1, 5, 6, 7
Scalenes	5, 6, 7
Pectorales	1, 5, 7
Latissimus dorsi	1, 5, 6, 7
Diaphragm	1, 2, 3, 4, 5, 7
Abdominals (3)	3, 4, 6
Rhomboids	5, 6
Glutei (3)	2
Sacrosoinales	4, 5, 6, 7
Ilio-psoas	3, 4
Iliocostals	4, 5, 6
Other Paraspinals	4, 5, 6
Intercostals	Deep breathing with 1 through 7
Diaphragm	Deep breathing with 1 through 7

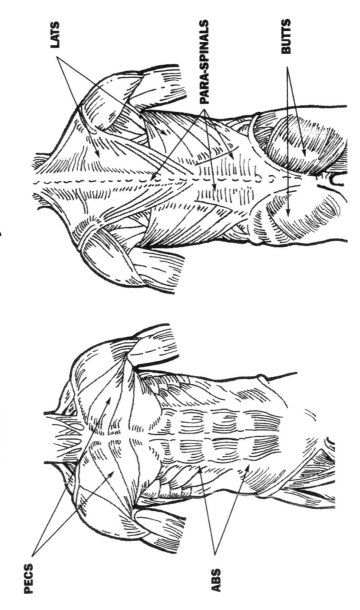

Figure 5.

Exercises are designed to stretch and strengthen these muscles and to move the joints they govern.

Chapter 7 ——————————————————
THE VALUE OF DAILYNESS

Throughout this book I have stressed the daily requirement part of the SEED formula. But its dailyness needs more than a casual inclusion; it demands a major emphasis.

For SEED to attain the status of a population-wide family habit, it must begin with a mandate for performance every day without fail. If it is presented as just another option to be added to other beneficial options, it will fail to become a real habit of action and a habit of thinking.

Habit stems from daily performance. The habitual aspect of SEED is what gives it power. As practice becomes habit, the small movements of progress build each day from a stiff, painful, awkward lower back to a supple, pain-free, freely functioning back. Little by little, each day builds on the last. Any daily slippage stiffens joints a little and serves as a set back. If you take one step forward you take two back by any omission. Each day's advance gives a platform for the next day's progress.

When you feel little twinges in your muscles, or when you don't feel as much improvement as you thought you should, just continue the daily routine. Don't quit for these reasons. It isn't much trouble to continue. In a few days what you thought was no progress will be forgotten as new mobility and freedom to function better while upright begin to appear.

Then after several years of performance you will realize that you have the mindset of a good new habit. You will miss it if you don't do it. You will trust it to pull you out of daily "low" moods. You will reflect on it, in pausing during a hectic day, as a sure-fire reviver for flagging physical energy and mild depression. I do it in the late afternoon, but it can fit into your day at any point that you find suits you.

Such is the power added when SEED finally becomes a habit. At this stage it really constitutes a permanent restorative factor in your life that will surprise you.

If you feel too busy for SEED on certain days, that feeling confirms that you need it all the more. If you feel that the mere performance of 13 minutes of SEED is hard work, that also confirms that you need it more than most who do it easily.

Never omit doing SEED each day. No excuses for Sundays, holidays, traveling. Those occasions are just lazy excuses. SEED will invigorate you and you will feel better particularly when it becomes a habit. Habit comes from never omitting it from your daily routine.

Chapter 8 _____
MY EXPERIENCE WITH SEED

During the last 20 years I have developed a whole host of diseases; any one of these can have lethal complications. I've had good medical care, meaning prompt diagnosis and the use of standard medications and other treatment. So far I have survived well, whereas most of my contemporaries with similar troubles have succumbed. This surprises me. Medical care is good, but I didn't think it was good enough to take an ordinary human being through an extra 15 or more years in good functioning condition in the face of gout, arthritis, a persistent heart irregularity, chronic lung disease from 47 years of cigarette smoking, large intestinal diverticulosis that threatens severe complications, stomach regurgitation, prostate gland enlargement, kidney stones, cataracts on both eyes, hearing loss and memory lapses. I have had six operations in older age with general anesthesia. I seem to have had everything except cancer and a stroke. Everyone of these conditions progresses in most people in my age group to the point of destroying normal functionability that leads to an early death. Not so with me. So far, these conditions have remained "on hold" for a decade or more at least.

Why hasn't gout given me such pain attacks as to make me an invalid? Why hasn't my heart given out, my lungs quit functioning and gone into terminal pneumonia, my large bowel bled or ruptured, my prostate developed cancer, my eyes gone blind, etc?

No one can answer these questions. Good luck merely means life is naturally chaotic. Good medical care helps, to be sure, but others have it also. Good genes? No one has been especially longlived in my family. Good living habits? I was an addicted cigarette smoker and always drank alcohol with friends, never dieted. I stressed my body-mind in competitive work, in war, in a surgical career and in constant occupation. Pretty ordinary stuff, really. The only thing different in my life has been the performance of SEED for the last couple of decades.

Lets look at SEED performance in more detail:

Doing SEED means setting aside 13 minutes each day, getting down on the rug in the bathroom or bedroom and concentrating on bodily functioning. It gets to be one of those things like brushing your teeth, bathing, dressing. It is an everyday habit. You plan to fit it into your day where it fits best—on first arising, before lunch, after work or at night before bed. After a few weeks you do it automatically; you don't have to make it a big deal or worry about it. It's just one of those living routines you plan to do for the rest of your life.

SEED wasn't a burden to me because I was experimenting to help back pain. But after awhile it gave me a recovered feeling when I was tired, or thought I was getting a cold or a sore throat. Then I came to regard it as a sort of a medical treatment for whatever ailed me. It made me feel better. I began doing the exercises more fully and carefully; then I felt more recovered and relieved. When I was through the 13 minutes of routine breathing and moving, I felt ready for another day. The "day", of course, would be mostly sitting, when you analyze it physically.

SEED was somewhat of a duty to me in the beginning when

I wasn't sure of finding back pain relief. But even when it relieved my pains I found it had become more than just pain medication. It had become a mild general rejuvenator, and it was certainly not a bother anymore.

Now I look forward to doing SEED. It is something I can depend upon. I find it easy to fit in 13 minutes somewhere during the day no matter how unexpected events confuse my schedule. Whenever I feel tired, depressed or uncertain about problems that sit on my mind, SEED performance helps me out. Is this my imagination? As I keep doing SEED, the results continue, even improve.

At first I would do SEED only once every two or three days. Then when it became more routine I did it every day. When I slipped back to skipping days I felt an uncomfortable stiffness, particularly in my low back; I felt I had regressed and needed to catch up. Doing it every day worked better. Now I am on the verge of doing it twice a day to see what happens.

Naturally in this process of working with SEED, I began wondering why such a mild, simple bit of movement was the one thing that regularly gave me such a lift each day. From the first I had explored in my mind the idea that civilized mankind had slipped into extraordinary inactivity by all the easing of heavy work and labor-saving gadgetry and leisure that we have become used to. Then I began seeing that the specific form that inactivity had taken in our world was the position of sitting for almost every waking activity.

The more I thought about what lifelong sitting at work and play does to us and to our bodies, the more convinced I became that the reason SEED works so well is that it corrects precisely what sitting upsets—our lower spines. Sitting all our life throws our lower spines out of line. SEED limbers the spine and realigns it. And once we get in proper alignment again, our whole upright functioning life revives as a matter of course.

Now that I've lived and done SEED for another five years since I collected these ideas, I am more convinced than ever that they make sense: 1) Joints oil themselves with serous fluid from tissues and blood to permit painless, frictionless movement of bone over bone; 2) Movement, not inaction, stimulates this oiling; 3) Inaction dries joints and stiffens them; 4) Stiff joints can be restored to painless action even after half a lifetime of abusive inaction; 5) Restoring painless motion and thus alignment of lower spinal bones revives normal posture to allow us to pursue normal daily functions. I've pondered whether this scenario is solid enough for popular airing and decided it definitely qualifies as correct, particularly since a couple of thousand other people find solace and benefit from SEED also.

Chapter 9 _____
WHO NEEDS SEED?

When I say that everyone needs SEED, I mean everyone who sits all day, and that means all of us. The ordinary things society is doing to recover from a life of sitting don't succeed in recovering our body-minds from the subtle damage of sitting. But not everyone knows this; not everyone feels in their bones the need for a recovery measure. The sitting populace has different yearnings from group to group and I must point out each one separately in order to define what part SEED can play in various lives.

Children

Children are not born knowing what is ahead of them. Today it looks to be a lifetime spent in the sitting position; this causes mid-life disability, obesity, and pains. These can be escaped by daily habit. Each child deserves to be prepared for it. The reason we haven't been teaching children this lesson is that we have not seen the sitting problem as a real problem until recently; we haven't thought about what to do to remedy it.

A case in point is another potential calamity that used to threaten but one we've known about: losing ones teeth early in life. We now know enough to teach children to brush their teeth and see a dentist. And so they do this all their lives because it was made an early habit. No big deal. Most now keep their teeth lifelong. Spine disability is the same sort of thing.

SEED, or something like it, needs to become a habit in each child's routine. Only in this way will they continue it throughout life and escape mid-life disability and the early dependency that stems from it.

It sounds like a large order—a new habit for every child. It also sounds like I know everything and have the authority to dictate sweeping behavior changes. I sound like Big Mother. Maybe it's from 50 years of medical practice.

It just seems like common sense to me. Children will not think it a big deal if taught at home and in school to do a few minutes of floor calisthenics each day. They will do it if they see their parents doing it; the same with school time set aside when all teachers and students alike do SEED.

Teenagers

Here's where the rebellion sets in. Here's where school routines play the largest role in instilling good hygiene into young lives, by teaching the facts by example. At present no set physical education program standardizes activity universally for all. Society stands at the crossroads; indecision prevails about what is best, what can be afforded, what things to compel and what things to leave to individual choice. And the rebellious urge of teenagers jumps into any weak chink in the curriculum armor. Children and parents will complain loudly if any compulsory "phys ed" gets introduced.

But you have to begin somewhere, and the earlier the better. Junior and senior high school students need a physical educational component taught every year about how a life of inaction awaits them; that the harm to back and mind accumulates as life goes on.

They need an example of what to do about it. Teenagers need to know that there is a remedy for it. They'll defy it in every way possible. But if the wisdom of those who have lived thoughtful lives never gets instilled in the young, society will continue to follow a mindless course of least resistance and more troubles will ensue.

Ages 20 to 40

In this span of life humans are at their peak of functional ability. Physically and mentally they handle the full load of work and play with the energy for the economic and social life of the nation. They function at full capacity with full strength and wit. At this stage they don't feel the need of anything as mild as SEED. They know they need activity of some sort; they prefer strenuous sports and workouts, aerobics, running, weight lifting. Women are busy with houses, child rearing, often with jobs and second careers; they just want rest. Few of these young adults see any virtue in minimal exercise; they seek maximal, sweaty exercise and quick results.

The main trouble with this frantic, tense group in modern society is they can't take the time to see what's ahead over the long haul. They can't imagine not feeling and reacting as they do at their peak. They feel that modern medicine and dieting will keep them from the early disability they see in their parents and grandparents. Not so.

Here's where the relaxing and refreshing benefits of SEED play best. Like yoga and tai chi or meditation, SEED restores a natural, more tranquil balance to the pace of everyday life. It revives one's mood to a more hopeful state; it enables young adults to gain better perspective on problems, quiets down emotional swings, helps regulate the tenor of daily life. It adds to adult life; no deletion of present activities need occur.

In the 20s, 30s and 40s SEED is a good answer to what ails people. But they don't know about it and wouldn't feel the benefit unless they do it for awhile. Added to their packed lives—only 13 minutes a day—say, in the late afternoon, they need not change any other events in their schedule. It will fit in. This is a life period when overeating is often at its peak. Food provides the easiest tranquilizer and respite from the daily grind. Strangely, if you do SEED you'll interrupt the "work-and-stuff" pattern. SEED restores a more natural rhythm to life so you can hear your hunger-satisfied signal easier and avoid automatically using food to "get through the day." You have to stop and really hear your body and mind speak to you for a short period. Because when you are rushing through life so fast your sleep period is not enough to get you back on an even keel to face the next day in good shape.

Over 50 to 65 years

As middle age begins, people may first glimpse the need for SEED. This age group still supplies a majority of the energy to fuel our society and economy, but daily demands and the work load begin to look heavier and heavier. Provision for old age begins to loom as a problem. Children may be out of the nest and on their own, but their prospects of making a bundle and putting the whole family on easy street seem remote. And there's the thought: will a person become old and disabled before his or her time?

In our present stage of ignorance about the troubles from sedentary life, 50 is a good age to begin SEED, if not before. People won't see its need or benefit much before this age even though they'd be better off if they did. Practically speaking, 50 years of age is when you begin to face the difficulty of recurring back pains, stiffness, failing energy and doubts about the future. Men and women over 50 in this day and age definitely feel the need of more activity in their lives. They go to gym classes seriously; they take up yoga, or some new sport or other like golf or tennis or swimming. They plan vacations with physical activity in mind. They suddenly realize that the daily demands of car seats, computers, television and seats at entertainments are taking a toll. But they need something quick, easy, cheap and dependable for a result. Such persons have embraced SEED—when they hear about it—with enthusiasm. And they continue it because it feels good and fills a deep need.

Ages 65 to 80

Most of the people who spontaneously responded to my offer in the newspaper were over 65, mostly in the 65-80 age group. They evidently are a segment of the populace who feel the desire for more activity but have not found a satisfactory answer to this need in what they often describe as their "declining" years.

Persons over 65 often have a degree of back pain or general arthritic pains and general joint stiffness that is so rooted in their backs that it will take strong measures to reverse it. Also in this period of life degenerative diseases begin their progress; when they are diagnosed they are often advanced and hard to cure. The success of treatment often depends upon a good innate body defense mechanism to maintain an arrested state or cure, or to prevent progression of disease if it has not been cured. SEED will need to be practiced faithfully for many months before real benefit accrues. But relief will begin to occur if one persists. Even a confirmed couch potato will improve in all the above mentioned aspects. I say this with feeling, not because I am a couch potato, but because my lower back was stiffened in an awkward reverse C-curve when I began. It took many months to loosen it up and correct it. But it did indeed respond and it now remains corrected.

My point is that older people do benefit from SEED. It is not too late, as many might think. The daily refreshing experience increases once your back loosens up and you find you can rely on the daily lift from good posture and easy, full breathing.

Over 80

Very few "over-80s", relatively speaking, can report on what helps in their advanced years. But over-80s are the most rapidly increasing segment of the population, and demographers predict they will remain a significant part of the economy and, I would hope, of society in the coming decades. As long as they maintain functionality they can continue to communicate on the internet, provide useful counsel in public affairs, take a role in community projects and social gatherings, and contribute to the financial and emotional stability of younger family members.

As an "over-80" myself, I can attest that we commonly remain effective if we are mobile enough to make the contacts and accomplish the logistics to play our role. We have to be independent, able to care for our housing, clothing, bathing, some travel locally, at least, and with enough energy to put together a productive day.

Today we have to plan on keeping flexible in body and mind, because lifelong sitting still will tend to freeze up our adaptable bodies and minds and force us into something like pitiful images of our former selves.

What has always been accepted by society as the inevitable "congealing" of old age can be overcome; I have discovered this personally. SEED can be the sparkplug for this process; it is the way to put zest back into your life.

All centenarians advise to "stay active." None can describe in detail how they did it themselves. SEED begins to supply some of this detail. Different age groups need SEED for different reasons; particular segments of society profit in different ways.

The Obese

Obese people find themselves in a special bind. They are afraid of radical surgery to bypass the stomach or to cut away unwanted fat. These surgeries carry long recovery periods and significant complications; of course they do nothing for innate body defenses.

Even though large amounts of excess fat make any exercise difficult, body movement is the basis for any serious start toward recovery, no matter how fat or at what age. SEED is the absolute minimum amount of exercise that can be envisioned to begin effective reversal of weight overload. It is an indirect approach to be sure, but a safe and sure one.

If an obese person finds a way to get down on his back by using chairs to hold onto or to push on, they can start to perform SEED. Perhaps they need others to stand by and help this beginning process; at first, helpers may be needed to get them up again.

Just trying to perform the various deep breathing and muscle contracting-stretching movements will help. The more one persists, the easier it becomes. Finally one gets the hang of it. Fat people have large muscles that are strong and capable of moving the extra fat loads; they definitely need use and practice through some exercise. SEED pays off better than any other movements, in time and effort spent.

The sit-ups (Exercise 4) require some reduction of abdominal bulk to sit up all the way. I exhale fully to let my own gut bulk push higher into my chest cavity. A fat person may not be able to get over mounds of abdominal fat to accomplish a sit-up. But anyone can make the effort to begin. This starts an abdominal muscle strengthening, and back muscle stretching and spinal joint movement that initiates eventual recovery. With repeated trials you'll improve. Use the Exercise 4-A help. Don't accept anyone's defeatist remarks like, "You can't do it, so don't try."

Of course, weight loss is the obese person's goal. And SEED doesn't do much for extra caloric expenditure. But, as I have stated so often before, the habit of paying attention to the body's motion and action translates into heeding your appetite signals and to begining to lower caloric intake.

Obese people will need a lot more than SEED, but without SEED other measures may not work or sustain the progress you make. SEED is a starter, at least, and once begun it becomes highly worthwhile to continue indefinitely. SEED provides as good a base program for the obese as for any other group.

Most people in America are overweight. And most people reject the character defamation associated with "obese", so most of us who qualify as overweight by official medical standards resist being called obese. But many of us really are fat and would profit from admitting it and getting down to brass tacks about the matter. SEED is a starter and a continuer.

Athletes

From what I have described about SEED so far you would assume that naturally athletic persons would have no interest in such a minimal exercise routine. But I find quite the opposite.

The older an athlete gets, the more life's sitting routine causes stiffness every day, if not back pain. Periodic games and competitions and workouts never prevent this tendency of the body to freeze up and to need loosening. The older we get the more pronounced it becomes. Athletes all have been taught by trainers in college or elsewhere which warm-ups they must do. They all vary. Which ones are best for all athletes? Each athlete believes his sport needs what his coach or trainer prescribes.

The most important consideration for any athlete of proficiency is balance. Natural good posture that goes with muscular coordination forms the basis for a good athlete's performance in golf, tennis, baseball, football, basketball, or any sport you can imagine.

Some are born balanced, with perfect Greek-god posture. Some achieve it, some learn it, some recover it after losing it. If you can keep your balance while carrying out the athletic maneuvers of any sport, you'll excel and improve. Watch the champions; they are expert at keeping balance. Jack Nicklaus, Hale Irwin, Tiger Woods, Andre Agassi, the Williams sisters, Johnny Unitas, Michael Jordan, all are superb athletes and would be champions in any sport they chose. All have superb balance.

You may reply that they were lucky to be born with good balance. But that's not really an accident of birth. Look at three-year-old children; they stand just as erect as a tree trunk with weight perfectly distributed on legs so that the most relaxed position is the erect one. No effort is involved. This frees up their arms and legs to do anything they fancy, even when moving. They learn to walk and run similarly balanced. That is natural to humans. Now, however, the sit-down, high-tech age has arrived.

Though born balanced, we lose it by lifelong sitting requirements—but we can regain it. That's what SEED is about — regaining posture and balance. You would think that the process would be done standing up, but if the damage sitting does it mainly to stiffen the lower spine, then lying down begins this loosening up in the best way.

Mature athletes get stiff during a day in college classes, jobs, travel. They need a quick, sure start to regain posture and balance.

All athletes, particularly golfers, profit from using SEED as their warm up for this one basic reason.

Women and Pregnancy

There's no essential difference between the genders as to the importance of balance or the tendency for lifelong sitting to freeze up the lower spine into an abnormal curve. But child-bearing imposes a physical burden on women, a burden that men don't have.

The damage of stretching abdominal muscles, weakenening them and thinning them by the bulk of the fetus in utero, needs a lot of rehabilitation and recovery time to return the muscles to normal. Women seldom take the time and effort to fully recover. Doctors usually give post-partum rehabilitation a lick and a promise; then multiple pregnancies compound the harm and effort needed for recovery. After several full-term pregnancies most women get fat around the middle and don't do sit-ups easily for both of the reasons of adipose tissue and muscle weakness. Women have most trouble doing Exercise 4. That is the reason for 4-A; it is a device to prevent women who have had children from just giving up. They need it more than any other group because their abdominals are weaker than other people's.

My wife has borne three children to term and had all the usual complaints and difficulties when starting SEED. She persisted and used various versions of straps and pulling on her legs to accomplish the sit ups in Exercise 4. Now she does them in regular fashion; she is proud of her flatter abdomen and increased abdominal strength. Of course she proudly stands erect after each session to show how she has benefitted.

Disabled Persons

Not many people with serious defects in their anatomy, like spinal fusion victims or joint replacement patients, have reported on their SEED experience. Several with hip replacements do all the exercises except No. 5, and do them without trouble.

SEED is really minimal exercise, done almost always lying

supine (on your back). As such the only contra-indications to its performance would be pain associated with the contractions of torso muscles because of recent surgeries, or undue strains on weakened tissues from injury. Anyone who has fears on these matters may be advised to consult with their physicians before beginning.

The mild nature of SEED, compared to aerobics, running, etc., make it a good candidate for many disabled people to begin recovery. Post-surgical patients can do the deep breathing and stretching in bed very often by themselves; this resembles the usual recovery measures surgeons advise their patients to use. Patients who have had limb or head operations can do most of SEED immediately. The worst impediment to post-operative return to normal is the post-anesthetic lassitude and the mind-set that one must remain very still to let nature heal. Both retard recovery. The quicker that movement returns, the better.

People with leg or foot troubles often take to their beds or chairs for long periods; the elevation of the leg helps circulation and healing. But the prolonged sitting or lying compounds the muscle weakness and spine stiffness we all have from sitting and sets people's general fitness back even farther than normal sit-down living. Some parts of SEED are always advisable.

On the general question of fitness, let us remember to break it into its two divisions: recovery from general inactivity, and recovery from the specific back distortion from lifelong sitting.

Chapter 10 —————————————————————

MEASURING SEED PROGRESS

The longer I have continued performing SEED, the better I have felt. I have already described the many aspects of my increase in well-being. Always athletic and active compared to most people, I had unwittingly allowed my back to become quite stiff during my working years. Therefore, it was only after the age of 70 that I first began to focus on lower back mobility. In spite of athleticism, I had obliterated my lumbar lordotic curve to a fixed, abnormal position that was hard to correct. I began with a marked deformity that I didn't know I had; consequently I was in for a long correction period, although I didn't know it when I started.

Younger persons would not have that hardship quite as pronounced as I had. They would not be so inflexible in their spines; their sitting habit would not have "cemented" their joint spaces so firmly in so unfit a way. And so I predict that persons beginning SEED in their 30's or 40's would quickly gain full flexibility benefit and maintain nature's more or less normal state so long as SEED continues. Measurement of SEED benefit in young person's cases would show improvement in the first few months.

SEED is a minimal exercise program. It is not aerobics, nor a sports-fitness necessity, nor even a moderate exercise regimen. It cannot be thought of as, or adopted for, endurance training. It will not produce quick weight loss; it does not accomplish muscle building.

SEED is first and foremost a specific correction for the critical damage that sitting inflicts on the lower back. It does not show popularly pursued changes in weight loss, endurance achievements, or registered improved metabolic equivalent scores. It focuses on the lumbo-sacral angle and the mobility of the lower back so essential to good posture and functional performances while moving upright.

I have carried out several simple studies in the laboratory that any student could do in order to place SEED into a formal scientific context.

First, I measured caloric expenditure. Doing the seven simple movements in 13 minutes expended only 32 calories. That amounts to minimal activity. Even if I did that twice a day, I would only use up energy equal to moderate walking for half a mile or so.

A pilot trial study was carried out by the Sports Medicine Department of the University of Louisville School of Medicine to measure any change in muscle strength or joint mobility. The volunteer sedentary subjects had no back pain at the time, so I was not measuring pain relief. (Such back pain relief had already been experienced by many SEED practioners including myself.) After two months of SEED, sedentary people aged 35 to 55 showed only slight gain in back-attached muscle power. However, they did consistently show increased low back mobility. They needed this change and they got it. Back suppleness is restored by SEED.

Other benefits from SEED could be measured but these have not been done. We could measure change in posture and balance in walking, bending, etc. We could measure weight loss or weight steadiness over a year or more in time if diet and other activities could be controlled. We could compare golf scores over a year's period with other confounding factors controlled. We could study happiness levels and progression rates of specific chronic diseases over the years. Perhaps we can persuade younger investigators to do these researches, but they would need many years to complete.

If some doctors and other skeptics insist on evaluating the results of these prolonged clinical trials before agreeing to recommend SEED, they would condemn society to a long spell of the medical status quo.

Chapter 11 _____
QUESTIONS AND ANSWERS

1) WHY ARE THESE EXERCISES BETTER THAN AEROBICS OR GYM WORKOUTS?

The SEED program has a different purpose: to establish a daily lifetime habit for everyone to solve the daily damage of continual sitting. Aerobics and gym workouts address specific problems, like cardio-pulmonary conditioning after heart attacks, or for cardiac surgery recovery, or for rehabilitation from various chronic diseases like excess cholesterol, high blood pressure, obesity etc. Gym workouts correct arm and leg weaknesses and excess weight problems. There is certainly overlap with the SEED program; workouts help but don't fully correct back weakness and inactivity damage.

2) WHY DOESN'T WALKING DO THE SAME THING AS THE SEED PROGRAM?

Walking doesn't particularly strenghten or mobilize the back.

It certainly helps the general activity problem and is the easiest solution to suggest for most people. But walking is not focused enough to correct back stiffness and weakness from a lifetime of sitting. Of course, people should do both. Only the SEED program is easy for all persons everyday.

3) WHY DO THEM EVERY DAY?

Three reasons: 1) 1 have found my own performance of various schedules that I want to do them every day. On days that I skip, I wish I had done them. 2) Habit of doing any necessary healthy program daily, like brushing your teeth, only gets ingrained if done every day. 3) I've learned that 13 minutes a day is a minimum for sitting damage repair.

4) CAN I OMIT ONE OR TWO EXERCISES THAT SEEM DIFFICULT OR CAUSE SLIGHT ACHING?

We all need to do the full seven exercises to get and keep strong supple backs. When you begin them, certain exercises may seem difficult in some way. I urge you to persist in trying to do them all, perhaps in fewer repeats for easier sequences at first, until you get the hang of it.

5) IS IT IMPORTANT TO DO THE DEEP BREATHING RHYTHM WITH THE EXERCISES AS INDICATED?

Yes. See Chapter 12 on the importance of breathing.

6) IF I FEEL PAIN WHEN BEGINNING ANY ONE OF THESE EXERCISES, SHOULD I STOP?

Not entirely. Just ease off on the effort and extent of that particular exercise. Do that one gently so that the discomfort is minimal and continue at that reduced level until it becomes comfortable. Continue with the other exercise in spite of pains with one of them.

7) WHAT IF I HURT MY BACK? SHOULD I DO THE EXERCISES?

You need two weeks of relative rest of the muscles and ligaments that have small tears and bleeding points from the strain. They heal by absorbing the small spots of blood and laying down scar tissue. Things that help this healing are heating pads, massage, etc. Celebrex@ and other non-steriodal, anti-inflammatory pills help the pain. If you want to consult your doctor, by all means do so and show him the summary sheet of the SEED program. During this healing period move only so you don't hurt a lot; let pain be your guide to movement. But don't lie still in bed all the time. Absolute rest 24 hours a day won't speed healing and may delay recovery. After two weeks or so begin the exercises gingerly, say half the volume, slowly, but increase each day despite mild discomfort until you resume full performance daily. Keep in mind that resumption of SEED is your best protection against a repeat of the injury.

8) WHY NOT SOLVE THE SITTING PROBLEM BY STANDING UP FOR MUCH OF OUR WORKING HOURS?

The logistics would be impossible. Redesigning work places and attitudes would be impractical; the strain of standing for eight hours would cause complaints of tiring and people would quit at half time. Most pleasures depend upon sitting; people will not allow infringement on pleasures.

9) WHY NOT DO THE EXERCISES TWICE A DAY IF THEY ARE SO GOOD?

Why not? Maybe this would be better for some people, but I have not yet tried it. Once a day has proven perfect for me.

10) WILL THE EXERCISES HELP LOVE MAKING?

Yes. A strong back is a great asset in the action two people make together during the height of passion. Nothing shuts down the pleasure of passion like a pain in the back. You need some physical confidence to enter into fulfilling loving.

11) AT WHAT AGE SHOULD PEOPLE BEGIN THE SEED PROGRAM?

In grade school and at home I was taught to brush my teeth. I have kept my teeth with dental help. It would seem sensible to begin a similar health habit early to keep a useful back into older age.

12) CAN I ADD MY OWN EXERCISES TO SEED?
Yes indeed!

13) HOW CAN YOU STATE THAT CHRONIC DISEASES LIKE SOME CANCERS ARE PREVENTED OR DELAYED BY THE SEED PROGRAM?

Three lines of evidence support my statement: 1) Dr. Paffenbarger and other epidemiologists have accummulated extensive data that exercise in general delays or prevents breast, colon and some other cancers. No exercise studies show the opposite. (These investigations cover 40 or more years involve 45,000 college students.) 2) The application of the general principles of biology, and modern lab discoveries in molecular biology, reveal that for most destructive processes in nature there exist contrary activities, built in, that cancel these decays. If we can maintain physiologic balance in our bodies, we allow the life-prolonging processes to counteract the life-shortening ones. 3) At 87 I seem to have delayed whatever will get me in the end-—stroke, heart failure, cancer, diabetes, for example. Maybe I even have prevented them, and death will come from unanticipated ills. If I attribute this to exercises like SEED rather than luck, God, or inheritance, at least you must admit the weight of evidence is on the side of exercise. At least exercise is in the mix of possibilities, and exercise has the advantage of being under our control.

13) WHICH GENDER GETS THE MOST BENEFIT FROM SEED?

Women seem to benefit most from the feed-back that reaches me so far. They need them most from the back weakening from child bearing; probably women have a more natural tendency to care for their bodies than men do. But I must say men are also learning to do back conditioning and to recognize the spin-off gains.

14) WHAT DO YOU SAY TO SOMEONE WHO COMPLAINS, "I CAN'T DO SEED; IT'S TOO HARD?"

You are in worse shape than anyone would guess. If you don't begin SEED now you will soon be a victim of early degeneration. It gets easier to perform as you persist.

15) WILL DOING SEED HELP HANGOVERS?

Yes. SEED speeds metabolic exchanges that rid the body of toxins and speed recovery in tissues like the brain.

16) WILL SEED HELP WEIGHT LOSS?

Yes, but slowly. First expect stoppage of weight gain. A day of SEED expends 40 calories. This is not much for weight loss, of course. But by doing SEED every day it adds up over the month; the adjustments for fitness in your body help your awareness of real appetite, and that prevents stuffing too much food into your body. SEED is my daily habit and I eat whatever I want and keep a healthy weight. The key to achieving weight loss is learning to listen to your body's needs and learning to feel uncomfortable outside them.

Chapter 12 ─────────────────────
BREATHING AS EXERCISE

A close friend, of my same age and degree of functionability, told me once that his father had always advocated deep breathing as a key to a long life. When his father died at the age of 98, my friend said he found a printed sign on the outside of his father's roll-top desk that said, "Remember to breathe deeply." His father died because he was, in his own words, "tired of living", not of any specific degenerative disease. He seemed to have run out of energy at the age of 98. He had been a good golfer and a champion bridge player and was very active socially. His son is now 87 and believes his father's advice—he practices deep breathing every day, along with moderate walking as his only exercise.

This story occurs to me often as I do the exercises myself. I am perhaps overconscious of the breathing part of existence because I myself have chronic lung disease from years of cigarette inhaling; I cough a lot. Could it be that breathing is the key function of our bodies that controls the health of most other functional systems? As I keep studying aging and bodily degeneration and exercising as a conditioner, I am increasingly convinced that this may be true. Maybe it's even obvious to real students of biological systems.

Of course, oxygen fuels our bodies and minds; it gets to our tissues and organs via the blood circulation to give energy for all actions and functions. Anything that interferes with oxygenation threatens our vitality. We get oxygen from breathing.

It seems apparent to me that a lifetime of mainly sitting while awake would wind down the full efficiency of our respiratory apparatus to a level needed only for minimal existence.

More and more I picture the role of exercise as one of re-invigorating our flagging breathing capacity to re-energize our bodies and minds. Perhaps that is the way any exercise of whatever kind helps us; it restores the full energy level of our tissues by the full breathing we do. Perhaps this is why research studies show that the more exercise we do, the deeper and longer we breathe, and the fitter we become.

This simple connection between the amount of exercise and benefit has real limits, however. Few of us, comparatively speaking, can do strenuous exercise for a variety of reasons. Age, obesity, pregnancy, work duties, time and illness restraints, and many other things prevent us from being a nation of daily aerobic performers all our lives.

This line of thought is what confirms to me the value of a short, free, at-home exercise routine that everyone can do, and that contains a full breathing component in each exercise to achieve its effects. If this is not enough to give full aerobic fitness, at least it may be enough re-energizing of tissue to overcome the deadening effect of daily sitting-inaction.

If this is so, maybe just deep breathing at intervals each day would do the same thing. It's possible that it is so if my good friend and his father so benefited. Further knowledge of breathing suppression could come from research studies. I would love to be young enough to take part in them. It seems safe to assume breathing suppression is a widespread phenomenon in modern life and to assume that some simple corrective action, while awaiting scientific corroboration, would pay off.

A free and unobstructed circulation is the other main pathway to bring the energy of life to our body-minds. I constantly remind myself of this. The heart and arteries are tough adaptable organs that don't obstruct easily; the veins and lymphatics, however, are thin and compressible and subject to a slowing of flow and blockage by postural changes. The things we can do to improve circulation don't equal, however, what we can do to increase breathing volume. Vigorous exercise and minimal exercise both improve circulation but the change in respiratory exchange that occurs when we switch from inaction to exercise seems the more pronounced. SEED beefs up both breathing and circulation. Both are vital and work together.

Chapter 13 _____
ON BACK PAIN

Some wag once said, "Human nature is very prevalent." So is back pain. It bothers almost all people at times. It plagues half of all people in their 30's and 40's. It is so universal a complaint that "Oh my aching back" has become the common daily lament of most individuals over 50.

A 1999 medical textbook published by the Oxford University Press states that low back pain (LBP), which accounts for almost all back pain, can be documented as follows:
1) 18-26% of the general population has low back (LBP) at any one time.
2) 45% have an attack of LBP each year.
3) 80% have LBP at least once in their lifetime, enough to incapacitate them for one month or more.
4) Most recover temporarily; 2-3% never recover.
5) Almost all LBP is mechanical, not due to diseases as such (like

rheumatoid arthritis or ankylosing spondylitis) and thus is correctible.

About 20 years ago I began looking into back pain for myself, and found that the usual medical explanation of the cause of back pain—"wear and tear"—was becoming outdated. I found that conservative measures of treatment were many and varied and that no single one of them was helpful to everybody. Then I found at least one modern authority who suggested excessive sitting as the cause of most low back pain (Anderson).

Further description of how our spines evolved and performed in walking while upright revealed the insight that "the health of the spine should benefit from movement because nutrient-bearing fluid, that is essential for joint and bone health, is pumped when the joint is exercised." (Anderson) Immobilized joints tend to lose fluid. More analysis by Anderson concludes that walking should be encouraged "with ample movement of the pelvis and spine" and that "in sitting and standing the maintenance of lumbar lordosis is recommended." (Lordosis describes the normal spinal curves.)

After I found the simple set of calisthenics that helped my back, I realized what I had learned: 1) Motion oils joints and prevents joint pain; 2) lack of motion of a joint promotes dryness, rigidity, pain on movement; 3) the lower spine needs to be kept mobile by movement, not stillness; 4) the most likely cause of lower spine pain (LBP) is the persistent stillness of the sitting position we assume throughout all stages of modern life; this lower spine is where sitting distorts nature the most; 5) the more we sit, the more we push the normal lumbar spine forward curve, which is put there to facilitate upright position and balance, into a backward, reversed curve and fix it there; 6) this reversal of lumbar curvature (though relatively slight and hard to see) becomes a fixed part of posture as sitting life goes on and thus throws us off-balance in later life whenever we get up, walk, or perform any function upright; 7) most of us have repeated back pains and get a permanent bent-forward, disabled condition of our backs prematurely; 8) I speculate that the prevalence of permanently off-balanced middle-aged and older people causes premature aging, disability, dependency throughout the whole populace; 9) SEED oils low back joints and prevents LBP, corrects posture, restores upright balance and functionability, which is thereby preserved by SEED's continuous performance; 10) 1 know from my own experience, and that of many others, that the low back pain scenario is reversible by adopting SEED, the sooner in life the better.

The role of good sitting posture in this scenario is one of helping to maintain the pain-preventive gains of SEED, while we sit day-to-day. If we correct the lumbar curve back into a natural proper alignment, we prevent further fixation out of alignment. The 13 minute daily SEED performance oils and keeps flexible the various spine joints needed for good pain-free movement. The point is that correct sitting posture alone, as helped by ergonomics and personal awareness of good sedentary position, will not produce a supple, healthy lower spine. Only focused exercise will do that.

X-Rays Don't Show Pain...

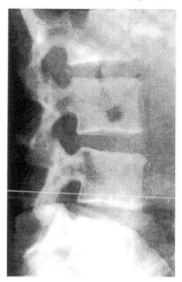 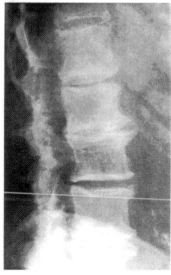

Normal X-ray of lower back
(young man **with pain**)

X-ray of Dr. Moore's badly degenerated
lower back
(Older man with **no pain**
who does these exercises)

Figure 6.

Chapter 14 _____
ATTENTION COMPUTER USERS

The most recent extention of sitting-abuse has accompanied the advent of the "cyber" age. We have experienced the sweeping injection of the computer into business and pleasure for less than a generation. However, every actively functioning human in developed society nowadays uses computers. It is a must in today's world. And, of course, we all have to sit still, crunched over for many hours, to do the necessary screen concentrating involved in computer use.

This sudden communications revolution actually increases the necessity of long-term sitting down. This sitting abuse is built into our computer lives now. It will surely increase in the future unless we correct for it.

Most computer users sit still while reading the screen, waiting for results, for E-mail to appear and for the electronic circuits to connect. The fascination with the ease of unlimited information available on all subjects, the world-wide breadth of coverage, fixes us all in a crunched-over position to get the most out of the system. And the more we sit and use it, the more we want to sit and use it. The E-world is a snowballing process in itself; computer use incorporates the essence of the sitting trap. It makes the message of this book a big part of the wave of the future.

The only thing that will allow the cyber-age to reach its full promise is a correction for the sitting abuse it requires. If we can develop a corrective habit to prevent sitting ailments, we will have it made.

This is what the SEED habit proposes to do. It restores the body's stiff back joints, muscle weakness and sluggish breathing and circulation. It does this each day after, or in preparation for, a day of sitting still. It restores the body-mind balance of ingestion-excretion, energy production and accurate brain wave circuitry. By this simple recovery habit, one gets more precise in one's observations and in making connections of ideas on the Web. By doing the exercises, at the end of the day one maintains emotional balance for relations with family and other people.

In my view SEED should be a part of every computer instruction manual, a part of introductory usage courses and a part of school computer training. In this way a sit-down life correction habit becomes a part of daily life.

Today's computer users are not old enough to experience the effects of a lifetime of sitting. The whole electronic world is too new for these consequences to emerge fully. But the physical impact is certainly coming in spades. Wise people should prepare for it.

Modern society cannot stupidly ignore what common sense tells us about the future. The day is past when we wait for an inevitable trouble to overtake us and say, "If we had only known."

We have a corrective habit that works. We must use it; or if we are critical of its structure, improve on it. We now know how to prevent sitting inactivity ailments. Let us simply inject this new habit into daily living and move on to the next important life problem.

Chapter 15 ———————————————————
IMPROVED GOLF WITH SEED

The tedium of explaining back pain relief in modern living needs some interruption now. The simple calisthenic routine I advocate has a lighter side: it definitely helps golf.

All my life I have been exposed to advice about how to play golf. My father was a senior champion, played constantly, practiced constantly, talked to me continually about how to hold your left am straight, to align your stance, to keep your eye on the ball, to swing smoothly and relax. All those things are important; all those things I practiced; all those things I tried to keep in mind with each shot. But I never got better than a handicap of about 16.

I love the game. I love the competition. I played sporadically until I was in my 50s and then began it more seriously. I read all the golf magazine instructions by all the experts. I watched golf on television avidly and found a key answer to my quest for the perfect game in a succession of champion golfers like Bobby Jones, Jack Nicklaus, Sam Snead and more recently Hale Irwin and Tiger Woods. I have also greatly admired the great basic swings and balance of women golfers like "Babe" Zaharias, Mickey Wright, and Annika

Sorenstam. Very little difference appeared to me in the ability to play golf between men and women; they were all great athletes, then became golfers.

I took lessons from a great club pro, Tommy Smith. I improved a little over a 15 year period, but I was no great golfer, I was just a great enthusiast.

Then I began doing SEED. This meant doing Exercise 7—35 shoulder turns a day. At first I felt that I was doing too many to help my golf; I was tiring out. But as time wore on the turns became easier and more natural and I kept my full turning arc over the years. As I did these 35 turns, I began thinking of my golf swing. I began thinking of keeping my head steady, which meant keeping perfect balance, which of course meant good spine alignment. After doing Exercise 7 I often took out a wedge, which I could swing on the rug indoors without threatening the furniture or my wife. I found I could turn fully and just brush the rug surface lightly with each swing, time after time. Wow! I'd never been that consistent and accurate before. I was not only learning to swing fully each time but I was learning real balance. I was learning not to bob my head forward by going up on my toes, a favorite weakness of mine.

Then I took my new shoulder-turn learning out to the course and found my direction and accuracy much improved; my "duff" shots were fewer and my distance was as good as I had a right to expect. I found a new sense of confidence that I now knew what to keep in the center of my mind on each shot—a full shoulder turn that I had grooved by Exercise 7, and the balanced stance which enabled a steady head.

Finally, when I stood over the ball on a golf shot I had the comfortable feeling that I knew what I was doing. Of course, I took careful stance in relation to the target; of course, I learned a simple pre-shot routine that led me to feel "comfortable" over the ball (as Jack Nicklaus often said); of course I took time to relax. No substitute for those things. But once I decided to swing, to "pull the trigger", I wasn't worrying. I could handle the two thoughts I needed to make good contact and get a reasonable result: head steady, turn from the shoulders while comfortably balanced; the rest took care of itself. The arms and hands and "body angles" and all the other body part adjustments that I had studied fell into line without my thinking. I learned to express all this to my grandchildren by saying, "I began grooving my swing" with Exercise 7.

This can't be the only way to groove your swing. Every good golfer has his own formula. Whatever works, works. But this one works better than the many magic solutions floating around today.

Today in my 80s I can fairly consistently hit a 3-iron 155 yards and drive it about 195 yards. I put together a respectable round on most golf courses. But I need a golf cart to save my energy for 18 holes. At 87 I'm considered unusual. This is mostly because I'm functional at my age, which most people are not. I shoot my age each year and have for the last 12 years.

PUTTING

The additional usefulness of shoulder flexibility, which has nothing to do with low back flexibility, surprised me when I applied it to putting. The more I concentrated purely on shoulder movement, to swing the putter, keeping hands and arms more or less rigid with hands perfectly still, the more accurate my putts became. Once I picked the line of a putt, the only thing I had to worry about, with my new-found confidence in relying on shoulder turn, was distance. It seemed to me if I could get the distance of a putt about right, I would seldom three putt. And this proved correct. My putting vastly improved.

No longer did I have to buy a new putter every year or two. No longer did I have to experiment with new putting grips. All my old putters and regular grips work all right now. True, I did switch to a reversal of hand position two years ago; that means left hand below the right. It helps keep my wrists from breaking.

Good putting is just about half of a good golf game. Watch any professional tour competition; the pro who is putting well usually wins. Why he or she putts well one day and not the next follows no rule. But consistency depends upon confidence in seeing the line and knowing the essentials toward getting the ball to follow it. My consistency has greatly improved by eliminating all movement except the shoulders.

Today I wouldn't think of playing even a few holes of golf without doing SEED first. SEED loosens me up, firms up my posture, restores a sense of complete balance and helps me remember how to play.

Every scratch golfer and pro has his or her own way of "grooving the swing." SEED works for me. Every pro may scorn moves other than his or hers. But whatever works, works. If you are not "grooved", try SEED.

Chapter 16 _____
THE EXERCISES AND SEX

Everyone knows love is what makes the world go 'round. While many kinds of love exist—love of things, ideas, spiritual devotion and platonic friendship—the heart of love is physical love, the appetite of lust and the actual bodily motions that produce and perpetuate the species. Physical love means sex. And sex perpetuates the species by being supremely pleasurable.

These fundamentals of human life have been minimized, suppressed and distorted as the organization of civilized living has progressed through the ages. Perhaps such a clouded consideration of sex was needed for civilized stability because the sexual appetite is so hard to control and so strong and uniquely joyful in its full consummation.

My conviction is that the attempt to limit civilized sex to procreative purposes only has failed over and over again throughout history. Why? It contains too much pleasure. Humans are constructed with too much natural appetite for sex to be able to control and suppress its performance to a few occasions when society sanctions it.

If sex for pleasure—the satisfaction of a strong, lustful appetite—is forced upon us by our healthy constitution, then it behooves us to seek health by satisfying our natural lust in socially stabilizing ways, lest wantonness produce chaos and ultimate self-destruction. This we do by the institution of marriage, and adherence to another human instinct—that of partnership fidelity. The human species needs both; the pleasure of lust and the fidelity of partners to build a stable family and produce responsible, maturing children who will carry on the race. We need both and we have both.

Whatever the details may be, the fact remains that men and women will pursue sex for pleasure for most of their adult lives as a natural part of healthy functioning. To reap life's greatest pleasure, whatever the ebb and flow of tides of love at various ages of life, both men and women require supple backs. This is one of the blunt and perhaps unattractive facts of life that refined and cultured societies avoid mentioning. Nice people don't talk about their personal plumbing, nor about sex, even though crucial decisions often revolve around them.

We can, however, discuss supple backs and their importance in a medical health context without fear of being "banned in Boston." And one of the joys of a supple back stems from the ability that pliable, pain-free backs afford to the enjoyment of physical sex. Nothing dampens the eagerness for sexual enjoyment more than an aching stiff back. Except perhaps a headache.

It is not my purpose to investigate the variations in people for the full enjoyment of physical sex. My main intent is to remind people that their full enjoyment of love depends upon the ability to please their partner.

Love is a unique pleasure in that it depends upon a partner. Half of love's pleasure is the joy given to the other person. Otherwise it is mere self-pleasuring greed and/or abuse of another person. You really cannot get the most fun out of love-making, give the greatest pleasure to your partner, with a sore, stiff back. When called upon to ratchet up the passion, you begin complaining or apologizing. It takes away half the fun. You may make do with half-way measures but you and your half-satisfied partner both feel the let-down when the natural impulses to make love fully are depressed.

After the age of 50 adults have spent so much time sitting still in life that their backs, especially low backs, are stiff if not hurting. By the age of 50 the stiffness becomes an accepted feature of "older age" and people adjust and make the best of it. My point is that it doesn't have to be that way. Backs can be kept painlessly mobile and able to function as nature intended.

You may misunderstand and think that by extolling the pleasure of physical love in the second half of life, when worries about unwanted child-bearing are over, I am favoring wantonness and promiscuity. Quite the opposite. I am saying that natural lust which engenders physical love-making can only be continually fullfilling with a partner. Partners may change, of course, over the span of a lifetime. But a real life partner is a hard-won prize, a fortune earned by constancy, intelligence, devotion—all those qualities that we learn to value. And luck must be a part of the picture, too.

If you value love, and we all do whether we know it or not, you owe it to your partner to keep a supple back. You owe it to yourself to keep the path open to satisfying physical love. Where love is concerned, half of it is your partner's pleasure. You give it to your partner because that is half of your own pleasure. You are not just averting pain by doing SEED; you are keeping faith with your partner. Don't let him or her down.

Chapter 17 _____
THE EXERCISES AS YOU TRAVEL

Traveling in cars and airplanes now occupies much of our waking time; it can only be done while sitting still, strapped in place, a behavior discipline that exerts a toll on us: weariness and back pain. Then we compound the damage done; when we reach our destination we resume the cramped sitting position in rooms, desks, restaurants and other meeting places.

When travelers undergo hours of inactivity they cannot be in the gym working out; or walking or swimming or otherwise moving their vital back joints. When travelers arrive at a foreign place their quarters are strange; they don't have their accustomed home surroundings with furniture and other amenities. They have to make do. And usually it seems too much trouble for most people to develop a time and place to do their daily toning up routine.

In order for SEED to effect its benefits in our lives it must

115

be done every day without fail. This is difficult when traveling. You don't make up for missed days by doing the exercises more energetically or more often when you get home; the stiffness of vital low back joints doesn't respond well to extra exertion to catch-up efforts. Extra SEED effort results in soreness and an enforced rest, which amounts to a setback. Joints need constant regulated motion to pump joint fluid into the joint spaces to allow pain-free motion.

SEED adapts to these travel situations remarkably well. Once you get out of your straps and restraints and into the hotel or motel room, all you need is a six foot square of carpet, perhaps a chair, a bench or a table, and a 5-foot broomstick; but the broomstick for Exercise 7 is hard to come by.

I have found that a folding cane made by Ambutech of Winnipeg, Canada, fills the bill for a traveling broomstick very satisfactorily. It is 50 inches long, comes in five sections of light plastic with metal fittings that are connected by a strong spring cord that snaps it firmly into place when put to use. It snaps out to a firm shaft and folds easily, when you are finished, into a one foot-long handy package that is light and can fit easily in any carry-on bag. You have it with you always when traveling so you don't have to worry about doing the vital Exercise 7 when away from home.

These folding canes will be supplied quickly upon request for $12 plus $4.50 for shipping. The address is 34 DeBaets Street, Winnipeg, Manitoba Canada R 2 J 359. Be sure to request the 5 section cane that measures 50 inches in full length so that you get a stick that suits the exercise.

If you are a frequent traveler you will get considerable satisfaction from having such a cane for use away from home. You will find that you will use it at home as well because it is so convenient and light and handy. It has lasted me through the years without bending or breaking because I'm not putting great stress on it. When I first began to do SEED, I couldn't find a suitable broomstick around my house. I had to go to Home Depot and purchase a 5-foot wooden dowel (5/8 in diameter) and fit it with a length of enclosing styrofoam insulation that is made to insulate pipes. This formed a convenient exercise stick that was soft on the shoulder and upper back when doing Exercise 7. I still use it at home.

You can't beat the traveling folding stick. The beauty of it is when you reach your hotel room after a long trip you have it available to begin SEED. I find that the tiredness after a long car or plane trip comes not from over-exertion, which you haven't done at all, but from the cramped-up, unmoving position you have been forced to take for hours at a time. The refreshing feeling you get from lying flat in bed partially revives you. But the performance of SEED has three times the restorative effect. After a long trip, if you rest and do SEED also, you have revived completely, ready for the meetings and festivities you have traveled so far to enjoy.

Travel Cane

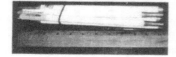

Collapsible cane in 5 sections (each section 11 inches long) held as a unit by strong elastic

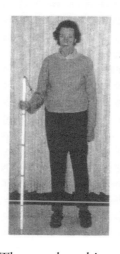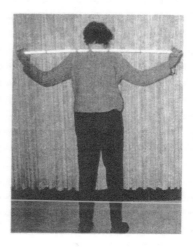

The travel card inserted in this book can be taken out and placed in your pocket or purse. Then when you stop for rest, or overnight, you have it for reference—a reminder of the sequence, the number and the procedure of each of the Seven Essential Exercises Daily. In this way travel need not delay your quest for back recovery.

Chapter 18 _____
THE FAMILY HABIT

A family that prays together, stays together. I propose that today we need another new family tie—a mind-body unifying activity that comes from preparing together, that is preparing each other in the family to have natural health, especially the children, to meet the threatening demands of the modern world.

The contemporary busy, demanding cyberage scene of today that we and our children have to face no longer falls under our control as it did under the constant religious faith which our forefathers had in their tight family units of the past. Previous generations found courage and support in an abiding, community-wide belief in God. Churches dominated community life. That support is gone, or at least greatly weakened. Religion as a life guide is now fragmented, questioned, or abandoned; the explanations are many but the remedies are obscure. Science and reliance on learning, on fact-gathering, on the study of evolution, don't promise comparable peace of mind and self-confidence for an entire populace.

Where do we go? We go to nature, is my suggestion. We must learn to know and feel the power of our natural endowments as humans; we need to learn how to maintain these powers and gain purpose in life from the miraculous healing and recovery mechanisms built into us.

Once we get this vision and feel the strength of the vision, we may gain enough confidence in ourselves to face the cyberage. When we gather and enlarge this vision together as a family, reinforcing it daily by a common activity, then the family and community vigor lost by waning religions can begin to return. We regain our purpose, our sense of identity and we can begin to rebuild our tumbling spiritual houses when we gain this new faith. Nature teaches us, if we listen. We have within our natural makeup this potential.

How do we begin such a family-type of preparation for natural health? The performance of some routine like SEED (and I have found none any better or as good so far) constitutes a real start. It is quick, adaptable to the whole family, costs nothing, and requires no scheduling or special locations or pain and suffering. It is not a conventional discipline of children, because parents enter into it along with the children. Preferably the family does it together just before breakfast each morning or before the evening meal at night. Parents show the children how and explain why, as they do it together. There is no exception for any reason except real illness. Children are told they must do this with their parents daily to keep from getting sick from all the sitting they must do each day. The car-culture, the school-culture, the TV-culture and computer-culture life leaves them no alternative. Children do SEED with the family or else they get no supper. It's not cruelty; it's necessity. Parents need it as much or more than children.

This can be a habit requiring no abstruse intellectual agreement or justification. It just makes sense. You don't do it because it keeps up with the Joneses or because the church or government advises it, or because you can save money and save taxes by doing it.

You just do it because the kind of world we live in demands it; it is like bathing, clothing, or brushing your teeth.

Children who can't understand the need for SEED will just have to wait to grow into such understanding; in the meantime they keep their parents company by doing SEED with them, waiting for breakfast or supper. Children who refuse or children who merely sit by and laugh or jeer at their mother and father will soon be bored when the rest of the family joins in doing SEED and ignores the refusenicks. Rebellious teens will have to go the way of other rebellious teens and mature elsewhere than in the family. But they will know how adults stay healthy in a life of all-day sitting and hopefully they will see the light in time.

When SEED becomes a family habit, argument and opposition disappear. Reasons for its benefits crop up in youngster's minds; they will begin to note how puny and lost their school friends appear whose families don't have this mind-body working tone-up. Soon they will begin to stand taller and show pride in their family and its habit.

Children will not feel the benefit of doing SEED in their bones like over-50 people do. Young people naturally have the good health and quick recoverability to avoid the stiffness, the lassitude and the back pains of sitting that adults all feel. They need parental example and family discipline; they need the force of having a habit and perhaps some peer pressure from their older siblings or friends, when SEED is done in families.

I am venturing out of my area of expertise to advocate such a social change in our culture. However, this projection becomes inevitable when one considers the implications of wide-spread usage of something like SEED. You have to wonder if SEED is suitable, if it is practical, if there are complications. You have to speculate on whether it will ever be acceptable to all persons. You have to ponder the alternatives.

When I try to imagine the universal usage of SEED as a family habit, I must confess it seems entirely workable, useful and promising. I've gotten it partly incorporated in my own family. I realize it takes time and patience and lots of explanation to begin with. But the end result with me so far has all been positive. Everyone in my family is happy with it.

True, the proof of the pudding will take years to emerge. I won't live long enough to know the end result. At least if SEED is tried it will prompt some people to develop something better.

If SEED evolved as a corrective for an established stiff, painful, out-of-line back, then certainly you would expect the same method could be a preventive measure if used in life before the back became fixed in a bad way. If young people did SEED they would never get in the pickle I found myself in at age 70. They would maintain supple lower spines all their lives to their great benefit. They wouldn't do it because it got rid of their back pain - they wouldn't have any. They would do it because it was an ingrained habit from childhood. Or because everyone they loved and respected did it. And it would pay off in pain-free, functional longer life.

Chapter 19
THE EARLY DISABILITY SYNDROME

The more I learn and ponder about the degenerative diseases (heart disease, cancer, stroke, etc.) that carry us off before our time, the more I view them as a single entity of degeneration that hits everyone to varying degrees, progresses with varying speeds in different people and destroys different organs in different persons, all causing disability to perform ordinary daily tasks, but with a common underlying control. Such a sweeping generalization can be picked apart easily by scientists and doctors. But I think it may help to find practical approaches.

A lifetime of inaction, which is what we essentially now lead, results in poor function of the recovery systems of our body-brain during waking hours. It allows "wastes" to accumulate in arteries, in brains, joints and in all vital organs. These wastes are not excreted or neutralized freely because, when we remain unbiologically rigid, still, crunched-over for long periods, our disposal systems become sluggish and inefficient. They need more motion and activity during the day to enable them to carry out their job.

More specifically, take heart disease. Most heart disease comes from poor blood supply to the heart muscle; this stems from waste material called "plaques" blocking small heart muscle arteries. The heart beats by the heart muscle contracting 70 or so times a minute; a full blood flow yields oxygen to give muscles energy for this constant demand. If something blocks this supply to the heart, the heart falters and fails. Plaques that accumulate in small arteries of the heart can block blood flow and become a vital emergency, whereas in our other organs arterial blockage doesn't threaten us with death so acutely when deprived of oxygen. These plaques are composed mostly of fatty compounds.

Two processes control plaque build-up and other waste accumulation: 1.) We take in too much food material and it overwhelms our bodies, disposal systems, or 2.) the disposal system is below par and doesn't process the food material thoroughly enough or fast enough. Controversy flourishes over which of these two pathways is faultier and which one deserves scientific attention and fixing first. Is it the intake or the outgo?

Medical research concentrates on the first pathway, the intake one where we eat the wrong things. By choosing this, medicine assumes that we all have properly working disposal mechanisms.

But what if our repair and waste excretion machinery isn't working well because we lead such indolent lives that disposal is rusty, creaky and inefficient? Wastes then accumulate even though we eat properly.

This is my proposal: consider the second possibility that medical research has not yet fully tackled; consider how we can bolster and revive our excretory, poison-neutralizing, healing, repair and immunity apparatus to meet the vagaries of the external world at least as well as nature provided.

A mountain of research studies each year reports that degenerative diseases are appearing earlier and progressing faster in people's lives; therefore death occurs earlier than should be. It seems only logical, when contemplating a reversal of this trend, to lump degenerations into a single category. Medicine uses the word "syndrome" for a set of symptoms that characterize a particular disease. I find it helpful to conceive of a new entity I call "Early Disability Syndrome". My use of the word "disability" comes from the fact that these degenerative diseases give us gradually increasing loss of function, which is what hurts us and what we feel and fear. Already doctors have coined the term "metabolic syndrome" to denote this same pattern.

The symptoms of Early Disability Syndrome would include obesity (high BMI-body mass index), back pain, arthritis, unsteady balance and gait, shortness of breath on exertion, progressive memory loss, other sensory reductions and a tendency to mental depression. The diabetic complex is also a part of these symptoms.

These complaints come from various already identified chronic diseases that medicine diagnoses and treats. People don't have all of these altogether at one time but the early-in-life onset (obesity in children for example), their persistent progression, one or some or all of them, their association with each other, makes me think that lumping them together will help to clarify a common underlying cause. If we can find that, then we might find a common correction or cure that would help all of these symptoms at the same time.

The diseases I think of as lumped together in a degenerative category are heart disease, cancer, arthritis of several kinds, adult diabetes, high blood pressure, the dementias, (especially Alzheimers Syndrome), stroke, obesity and general depression. Less well-recognized conditions may fall into the same category: the mylagias, the neuroses, several chronic vital organ failures; others such as multiple sclerosis, Lou Gehrig's disease (AML), attacks of vertigo (dizziness) and tinnitus can be so classified as well. Diseases classed as "auto-immune" and those called "psychosomatic" may fall into the degeneration category, or be caused by the same complex of factors.

Perhaps I am talking about chronic diseases in general. I

will not try to carry this generalization further; it will soon overlap with structural defects and genetically determined illnesses. Many scientists are seeking a genetic basis for every disease entity since the unravelling of the DNA structure. Tendencies to develop many degenerations from genetic differences are being found. But genes are only one factor in the combination of forces leading to the type and timing of most human demise.

If what I choose as a concept is justified, you will question why the average longevity of our population creeps upward a little each year rather than going downward. If early degeneration is advancing, the average age of death should be declining. My answer is that the medical advances in the last century have been so spectacular in acute and infectious disease-causing afflictions that they are slightly overcoming the chronic degeneration trend. One is cancelling out the other. And if it weren't for chronic degeneration we would now be, I feel, averaging a lifespan in the 80's and 90's.

The various diseases that I mention in the early decay group have characterized aging in all human eras throughout history. People have always succumbed to heart disease, cancer and the dementias if they live through acute ills and accidents and wars. We are not facing anything new in life, just different proportions of old things. How can we handle these early degenerations that so deprive us of years of later natural life?

I think we can begin by doing three things: 1.) Begin to see ourselves constituted to live 100 years or about that much; regard death before that time as preventable and search for ways to prevent it. 2.) Realize that death from the decay type of disease can be controlled to a meaningful extent by our own common sense living habits and good medical care; certainly they can be delayed somewhat, delayed ideally to 20 or more years longer than popularly assumed. When you acquire this viewpoint, which is the one I have finally adopted after 60 years in medicine, you gain real hope for, and perhaps a belief in, some such culturecorrective habit as SEED. 3.) Do SEED.

SEED may not be the final remedy but it is a start toward keeping all organ systems in harmony, toward balancing intake and outgo of foreign substances, toward "homeostasis", such that any chronic degeneration doesn't go into high gear and begin a cascade of organic failures before nature decrees it. By making this start you will be in position to recognize any improvements over SEED that are worthwhile. More important is the positioning of your future enquiries toward expanding the field of preventive medicine by discovering how best to bolster innate biologic defense forces. In this way humanity can double the benefits that medical care has already bestowed by curing or controlling specific organic diseases.

Chapter 20 _____
THE SEVEN EXERCISES AND AGING

Aging is another natural life occurrence, like hunger and sexual drive, that we all experience and talk about. As with those other forces, aging has to be accepted for what it is, not for what we think it should be. In the case of aging we imagine it as what we see happening every day in people around us. I believe that this popular view is not natural aging but is a combination with disease. (See Chapter 1.)

What we usually call aging, what we observe in our family and acquaintances, is the result of the combination of two processes: natural inevitable aging acting together with the widespread early chronic diseases that affect our civilized society. This latter process I've described in the previous chapter, calling it Early Disability Syndrome. Natural aging, measured in the laboratory by the number of cell divisions that mammalian cells undergo before dying out, can only be roughly estimated for a human being. We are composed of hundreds of types of different cells; but, as I've previously stated, 100 years of natural life is a reasonable expectation. We are actually dying in our 70's. So aging results from the early chronic diseases that we all have, acting together with natural aging.

A close look at aging makes us see it in practical terms: it is really a loss of natural human function. Ponce de Leon sought the "fountain of youth", the magic that would enable humans to function like 20-year-olds for a lifetime or more. It is functional decline that all humans have feared throughout the ages. We learn to expect a slow falling-off of our abilities to cope as the years go by; we learn that functioning is our main source of pleasure in being alive; we continually wonder what can prolong good function.

By human function I mean all of the physical, mental-emotional reactions to life that we are equipped to engage in so we can live. We have pleasurable feelings, hard wired into our human natures, that are connected to successful performance for functioning. Happiness depends upon good functioning.

What does function consist of? It is all the things people do and think. It is taking care of yourself each day without burdening others; it is observing accurately, dreaming, planning, empathizing with others; it is using a personal learned skill or natural ability to accomplish a task better than other people can. It is all these things and many more that I haven't the wit to list.

As we consider the society-wide life habits that could be charged with encouraging the early onset of chronic diseases, which is the unnatural component of aging, we cannot but conclude that sitting-inactivity heads the list. Sitting is far more prevalent than accidents, injuries, accute illnesses or environmental damage. ,

I've discussed in earlier chapters the reasons that the inactivity hurts us. You may disagree; you may fail to see how sitting all of our lives can harm us. No one so far has indicted sitting as an evil thing. Civilization has always regarded it as a boon and a reward and a rest from work. But I believe it is now being abused by overuse. I believe it is a highly reasonable hypothesis to connect sitting with early chronic disease. Furthermore, this indictment is not just destructive criticism; I have found a beginning antidote. If sitting is the culprit, we have a start at a correction. And while many readers may disagree, many more others agree that it makes sense.

The outcome from this view of aging amounts to doing SEED; everyone who sits needs SEED. Just as SEED starts us on the road to recovering our natural daily flow of repair processes which we have lost gradually during a life of sitting crunched over and unmoving, so SEED performance gives us hope of postponing unnatural aging and allowing the natural course of functional decline to occur in a more native pattern.

Two facts about aging enter into doing SEED. 1.) Only after the age of 50 do people feel the need for SEED; 2.) the later in life SEED begins, the less its effect in countering sitting damage and the longer it takes for the benefits of SEED to kick in.

When we consider these two facts, it seems intelligent to begin SEED early in life to get the most out of it. After all it doesn't require money, time or real effort. If we begin it in youth it will become a habit, part of our daily routine. Otherwise it entails learning a new routine in later life when learning something new is difficult and slow and often controversial; at that time it is likely to be discarded. We are fully addicted to an easy, entertainment-filled life; we are brought up to feel entitled to continual pleasure. Only if, early in life, we get used to a routine will SEED fall into place as the missing link in really enlightened living.

The secret to aging, happily it seems to me, is to preserve the ability to function in the way humans were made to function. If we have this functionability, we receive built-in pleasure from it. We are not depressed; we are not unhappy; we are not a drag on the minds of our family and friends. We take care of ourselves. Our loved ones are proud of us for being happily independent. Have you spoken to a relative of a fully functioning 95-year old recently? They speak of such nonagenerians with pride and enjoyment. They look forward visiting that "old" person, who inspires and delights them. No one hangs crepe prematurely for such old timers. Older functioning people contribute to, rather than detract from, the happiness of others. We are happy with them and for them.

Of course many oldsters have incurable or debilitating

diseases that preclude my happy story line. Many of them were not preventable by the age of 70. But, on the other hand, many debilities are reversible if caught in time. The seemingly innocuous feature of modern life that stands in the way of long-functioning life is the sitting feature. Sitting inhibits late life functionability. It is correctible not by eliminating sitting but by countering its harm through a daily new habit.

Chapter 21 _____
THE CASE FOR SITTING

Sitting is basically a good thing. It only becomes a trap from overuse or poor use. When we think about sitting, the distinctive good features of it can be listed as follo2ws: 1) We have to do it—lots of it —both for work and for play. 2) It's a pleasure. 3) Any harm from sitting is not obvious. 4) People have always enjoyed sitting throughout human history. 5) It appears to be as good as sleep for restoring our functioning powers.

With all these positive features in its favor, why isn't the human race made for sitting down, instead of being constructed to be erect and moving? Since evolution is the only natural designer of basic structure that we can be sure of, the answer to the question is that evolution hasn't had a chance to mold us into modern civilization's sitting predominance. Evolution takes thousands of years to effect major changes in a species through survival of the best adapted. Because technical-age sitting is so new, evolution simply hasn't had a chance to work. And by sitting design, of course, I mean both the design of our physical structure as well as the design of our functioning systems to coordinate with each other. Therefore, if we are not in possession of a sitting design we have to use our wits to adapt to our sitting, technical life today. The promising strategies which we are now using to bring about such adaptation are a.) Chair design; b.) Moving around in all sorts of sports and programs in our spare times; c.) Learning habits of good posture in sitting and standing; d.) Walking as the US Public Health Service recommends; e.) Using our medical care system to medicate sitting ailments. As I've discussed in previous chapters, each of these strategies has its pluses and minuses. They have been in effect long enough to have brought about what changes they are capable of and, as we have seen, are not only failing to solve the problem but allowing the problem to worsen.

To give sitting its due, let me take up the positive points about sitting one by one:

1) We have to sit. I agree and cannot suggest a substitute for sitting-inactivity. Sitting is a must to concentrate, communicate and travel in today's world. Therefore we need to develop a way to live without letting sitting-inactivity harm our total lives. We must be able to sit and not worry about it. The critical problem is how to live with it. This I am confident we can do and therefore the necessity of sitting as a positive feature cannot and will not be changed.

2) Sitting is a pleasure. We don't have to stop enjoying sitting. By "sitting-trap" I mean the trap of abusing a good thing. The way to avoid spoiling the pleasure of sitting is to devise ways to thwart the dangers of overuse. If we can devise some counter activity, like SEED, then we can continue to enjoy sitting as a pleasure without having to worry about curtailing it or changing the way we do it. Sitting is a reliable pleasure and will continue to be so.

3) Sitting-inactivity harm is not obvious. This is quite true until later in life. At the age of 50 we begin to experience that sitting still has ill effects; but we don't connect them to all the sitting we have done throughout our lives up to that point. We attribute those ills to "aging", poor habits in youth (probably partly true), inheritance or old injuries. Certainly most people think of these ills as irreversible.

Such a line of thinking and belief is mostly false and fatalistic. In our resolve to get the facts straight, let's at least see the full picture throughout a long life. Let us gain perspective. If we wait until the full frictions of constant sitting exert themselves it will be too late for any cure.

4) People have always enjoyed sitting. This is true, of course, and people will probably always continue to sit and enjoy it. It is resting and relaxing and serves as a relief from many of the woes of daily living. That doesn't mean it can't be overdone. Today we are overdoing it to our detriment, but since we must do so, some antidote for the overuse of sitting will be logical and welcome. The fact that the human race has always indulged in and enjoyed sitting need not and will not of course change. We simply need a way for modern-day cyberage people to continue to enjoy it.

5) Sitting should be a restorative position. Sitting *is* restorative. But the way we use it today results in the opposite of restoration. It yields sluggishness, stiffness and a resulting slowing of mentation when we overdo it. Sitting in a reclining chair for a short period certainly is restorative, without question. But most of us sit bent forward in a physiologically awkward posture, compressing internal organs and flow processes, drying out joints for 8-10 hours a day and more. That amounts to a destruction rather than a restoration. With the proper antidote, sitting can be restorative.

SEED can be the answer to making sitting a pleasure instead of another burden. When you get in the SEED habit you find, as time goes on, many imbalances in your physical and emotional and intellectual life begin to straighten out and return from the imbalanced state that was forced on you by frantic study and the cramped-up positions that proceeded in previous years. These abuses you easily tolerated in your youth; but after 50 or so years they begin to impair function. That's what increases your fear of aging. There is a lot of pleasure in sitting. Like in eating and in sex, the answer to getting the best out of sitting is not to cut back on it but to get it in balance. Balance is the key. Balancing excessive sitting with SEED performance fosters the pleasure without paying any price for it. Thus you can sit without worry.

Chapter 22 _____
MY PREDICTIONS

If modern medicine controls or cures major chronic diseases, what kind of life are we preserving the general public for? A life of early functional disability seems to be in store for most of us today. It doesn't have to be so, for the reasons that I have tried to outline.

To follow this line of thought, I cannot refrain from speculating about how much added enjoyable life would be given us if we could all maintain easy, upright mobility while pursuing our careers. By this I do not mean our careers must involve this position; I mean a lifestyle containing habits that will maintain our natural postural mobility.

To put numbers on the benefit would be unscientific and imprecise. But if you, the reader, have been interested enough to go this far in the book, you may have been tossing around in your own mind these same possibilities.

In Table 1 below I estimate how long people live today related to how long a daily period of sitting they average in their lifetimes. It shows that I believe the most active persons, like dancers and athletes, live longest. But that doesn't mean I'm proposing we all be dancers or athletes to live longer and better. I mean this is the way things are today.

In Table 2 I estimate longevity as it might vary with some commonly recommended activities, with and without SEED. You'll notice that the addition of SEED alone to any average person's lifestyle in the 50s should increase his or her length of life by about eight years. My assumption is that people will delay the advancing rate of the chronic diseases that will eventually kill them by that much time. Then, if they add such things as walking, ordinary mild dietary caloric restriction, and average medical care to the mix, they will gain another eleven years in longevity.

These figures represent averages. Individuals all have mitigating peculiarities and unusual diseases that affect outcomes.

Presumably, if a person cares enough about his fitness and sees the burden his old age might have on his family, he may adopt SEED, or some equally mobile posture maintainer. Such persons would also, during their 60s and 70s, begin daily walking, begin to restrict calories, and get medical checkups, since these follow naturally when people are optimistic about their fitness and the future. The average person, therefore, might stand to gain nearly 20 years of added enjoyable life when comparing ordinary sedentary existence to a more enlightened one.

TABLE 1
Estimate of Longevity Related to Sitting Time

Percentage of daily sitting time	Average length of life
95	75
75	80
50 ⎤ ideal physical fitness	⎡ 85
30 ⎦	⎣ 90

These figures are highly conjectural. An individual in a lifetime would certainly sit for different average times depending on age and lifestyle variations. The added longevity stems from the upright, active lifestyle that will obtain if people don't sit most of their working hours. For instance, a farmer or a hunter would sit less than half the day. This active, upright life tends to delay degeneration.

TABLE 2
Estimates of Longevity with SEED and other aids

General Population Without SEED

	Average age at death
Inactive	75
Walking one mile 3 x week	80
Walking one mile 3 x week plus low-cal diet	83
Walking one mile 3 x week plus low-cal diet vitamins, good medical care	86

Effect of Adding SEED

SEED alone	83
SEED plus walking one mile 3 x week	88
SEED plus walking one mile 3 x week plus low-cal diet, vitamins	91
SEED plus walking one mile 3 x week plus low-cal diet, vitamins, and good medical care	94

These estimates assume that 60% of the population is "inactive", an often-quoted statistic.

This Table assumes SEED begins between 50 and 60. Such exercises may add up to two years to the length of life for every five years of exercises performed daily. If people begin earlier in life, which I would favor, who yet knows how long the benefit would extend? I would venture to suggest that each year of SEED might add one year of life.

Chapter 23 _____
In Conclusion

After 17 years of study, I have learned some things about back pain:

1) The sitting feature of modern civilized life hurts people over time. It results in a stiff, out-of-alignment lower spine. Back pain and poor upright functionability result. Many other ills follow.

2) The spine stiffens because joints that are unmoving over time get dry and accumulate deposits. Only motion lubricates joints to avoid joint pain and allow easy motion. Constant sitting congeals the back structure over time, which in turn affects many functions besides posture and gait—breathing, circulation, excretion of wastes and possibly immune responses.

3) A condensed, short set of easy home calisthenics that limber the low back reverses this sitting damage. I call this SEED, for Seven Essential Exercises Daily.

4) SEED works because it focuses specifically on the lower back joints and attached muscles which is where sitting wreaks its havoc. Also, it works because it makes one feel better; it gives pleasure;

it easily becomes a habit. It works because it corrects each day's sitting distortion with an adequate correction.

5) As supporting evidence, thousands of persons have undertaken the SEED regimen. They universally find it beneficial and continue doing it.

6) The only other regimen that even begins to rival SEED as a universal remedy for sitting is walking. But walking only helps the inactivity phase of our sitting culture, not the back troubles. Millions of us walk every day, but the sitting-connected ailments continue to get worse.

7) SEED supplements, rather than replaces, the benefits of medications, a balanced diet with vitamins and minerals, and it doubles the efficacy of sports or workouts. I personally have settled on frequent walks, medications under my doctor, and I play golf. But the most important thing I do daily for fitness is SEED.

8) SEED suits every person in today's world. It fits male and female, young and old, rich and poor, the powerful and the meek, the able and the disabled. Everyone needs it because everyone sits most of a lifetime and everyone will feel joy in it. It is free and easily available.

The spin-off health deficiencies from sitting-inactivity are now dominating public awareness. Obesity, early disability and chronic degenerative diseases increase every year in spite of outstanding medical advances, dietary preoccupation and the popularity of "fitness" programs. The picture demands a totally new approach.

The SEED set of movements can accomplish for Americans the same body-mind conditioning that Tai Chi and Yoga accomplish in eastern civilizations. Those rituals arose in more religiously dominated social orders than ours. America is a relatively new dominant culture in the world; any societal corrective like Tai Chi or Yoga will flourish here only if based on science and technology, which are America's strong points. SEED is based on physiology; it is a technical correction for a necessary civilized habit, the sitting position, that facilitates modern living. SEED corrects for sitting so society can continue to sit for a lifetime without fear of spoiling a natural—perhaps 100-year—lifespan.

I picture the miracle of life on earth that eternally reproduces itself as the imponderable, inexplicable wonder of the universe. Belief in God and eternal life is based on this picture. The miracle of self-healing and defense systems built into humans to allow us to survive and thrive for millions of years far outshines mankind's medical inventions and techniques to enhance survival. Without this miracle of self-healing we would be doomed. If we impede self-healing we die early. Today's civilized living makes sitting-inactivity the dominant characteristic of our lives. Without a correction for the damage this causes to self-healing, medical science may make only a paltry future contribution to the survival chances of mankind.

Readings

Certain books and publications have stayed in my mind as I wrote this book:

Anderson, R., *Human Evolution, Low Back Pain and Dual-Level Control*. In Trevathan, R., Smith, E.O., McKenna, J.J., *Evolutionary Medicine*, Ch. 13, Oxford University Press, New York, 1999.

Blair, S.N., *Changes in Physical Fitness and All-Cause Mortality*. Journal of the American Medical Association, 273, No. 14, 1995.

Boaz, Noel, *Evolving Health*. John Wiley & Sons, Inc. New York, 2002.

Cannon, Walter, *Wisdom of the Body*. W.W. Norton, New York, 1932. (I read this in medical school; it is still a classic).

Cassel, C.K. *Use it or Lose it—Activity May be the Best Treatment for Aging*. Journal of the American Medical Association, 288, No. 8, 2002. (This whole issue is on aging.)

Cooper, K.H. *The Aerobics Way*. M. Evans & Co., New York, 1977. Ehrlich, Paul R. Human Natures. Island Press/Shearwater Books, Wash., D.C., 2002.

Erikson, E.H. *The Life Cycle Completed*. W.W. Norton, New York, 1978.

Finkel, T., Holbrook, N.J. *Oxidants, Oxidation Stress and the Biology of Aging*. Nature, 408, Nov. 8, 2000.

Fischer, J.E. *A Look at Britain's National Health Service*. Bulletin American College of Surgeons, Feb. 2003.

Kirkwood, T.B. and Austad, S.N., *Why Do We Age?* Nature, Vol. 408, Nov. 9, 2000, pp 233-238.

Korner, J. and Leibel, R.L. *To Eat or Not to Eat—How the Gut Talks to the Brain*. New England Journal of Medicine, 349-10, Sept. 4, 2003, pp. 926-928.

Krause, W.E. et al. *Effects of the Amount and Intensity of Exercise on Plasma Lipoproteins*. New England Journal of Medicine, 347, No. 19, 2003.

Mokdad, A.H. et al, *Prevalence of Obesity, Diabetes and Obesity-Related Health Risk Factors*. Journal of the American Medical Assn., Jan.1, 2003, pp 76-79.

Pinker, S. *The Blank Slate*. Viking-Penguin, New York, 2002.

Ridley, Matt, *Nature Via Nurture*. Harper Collins, New York, 2003

Sandy, L.G., *Sounding Board*, New England Journal of Medicine, 347, No. 24, 2002.

Paffenbarger, R.S., Jr. *Lifefit, Human Kinetics*. Champaign, IL, 1992.

Wilson. E.O., *Consilience*. Alfred A. Knopf. New York, 1998.